Y's Way to WEIGHT MANAGEMENT

SANDRA K. COTTERMAN

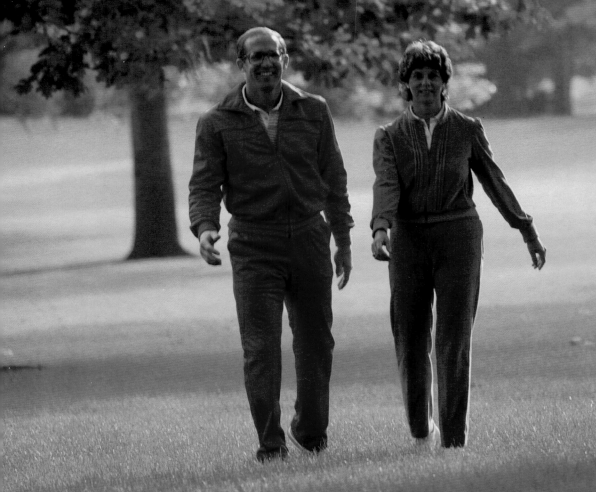

Exercise Log

The Exercise Log lets you see your weekly exercise progress and the number of calories used during exercise.

1. On the bottom half of the Log, fill in one block for each 10 minutes of exercise.
2. On the top part of the Log, fill in one block for each 50 calories you use while exercising.

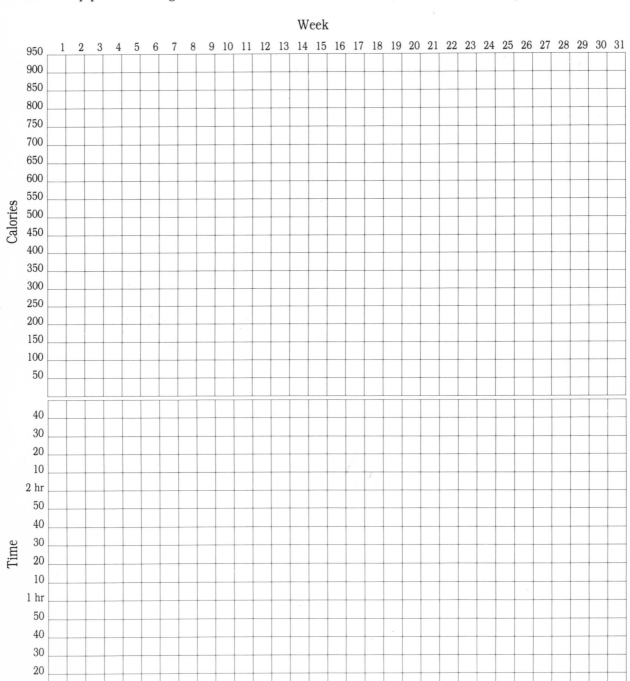

■Y's Way to WEIGHT MANAGEMENT

SANDRA KONRAD COTTERMAN, MS, RD
Nutrition Communications®

Developmental Editor: Gwen Steigelman, PhD
Copy Editor: Stephen Davenport
Production Director: Sara Chilton
Typesetter: Sandra Meier
Text Layout: Janet Davenport
Text Design: Julie Szamocki
Cover Design and Layout: Jack Davis
Cover Photograph: Larry Kanfer
Printed by: United Graphics, Inc.
Special thanks to John and Deanna Wright
Mr. Wright's clothing courtesy of The Tennis Partner, Champaign, Illinois
The National Board of YMCAs, The Vitamin Table and The Table of Minerals from *The Official YMCA Fitness Program.*
   Copyright © 1984 by the National Board of YMCAs. Reprinted with permission of Rawson Associates.

ISBN: 0-87322-032-3

Printed in the United States of America

6 5 4

Copies of this book may be purchased from the YMCA Program Store, Box 5077, Champaign, IL 61820, (217) 351-5077.

To my parents, William and Mary Konrad

Acknowledgments

Writing this program has been a tremendous opportunity to share my personal and professional commitment to nutrition education. My gratitude goes to Rainer Martens of Human Kinetics Publishers for his confidence in me and Jerry Glashagel of the YMCA of the USA for the chance to work with a terrific organization on a worthwhile project. My appreciation extends to the entire YMCA Wellness/Health Enhancement Task Force with special thanks to Mike Parks, Mike Ketcham, Medhat Mahady, Jo Ann Ploeger, Gerdy Weiss, Norm Joyner, and to Cliff Lothery of the YMCA who all willingly shared their insights for developing the program.

Special recognition goes to Gwen Steigelman of Human Kinetics Publishers for her efforts to bring the manuscript to press and to Barbara Schaffer of the YMCA of the USA for her administrative support.

I want to thank my loving husband and best friend, Bruce, whose encouragement and patience allowed me to undertake and complete this project; my daughter, Amanda Mary who at the age of 8 months would much rather have had the extra time to play with Mommy; my Mom and Dad for their love and guidance over the years and ongoing support throughout this project; and all my professional colleagues in the field who have worked so diligently to help nutrition education gain recognition and respect as an essential component for wellness.

CONTENTS

		DEDICATION	iii
		ACKNOWLEDGMENTS	iv
		WELCOME TO THE PROGRAM	1
Chapter	1:	INCREASING YOUR AWARENESS	5
	2:	MANAGING YOUR EATING TIME	13
	3:	CALCULATING ENERGY COSTS	23
	4:	DEVELOPING AN EXERCISE PLAN	37
	5:	MANAGING FOOD CHOICES	45
	6:	LOWERING YOUR CALORIES	57
	7:	MANAGING YOUR EATING BEHAVIORS	69
	8:	BUILDING SUCCESS TEAMS	81
	9:	MANAGING SPECIAL SITUATIONS	89
	10:	CONTINUING YOUR COMMITMENT	95
Appendix	A:	EATING AND LIFESTYLE QUESTIONNAIRE	99
	B:	ACTIVITY AND FITNESS BENEFITS CHART	101
	C:	NUTRIENT CHART	102
	D:	GUIDE TO FAT IN COMMON FOODS	109
	E:	CALORIE GUIDES TO EATING OUT	113
	F:	CALORIE CHART	121
	G:	REFERENCE SHELF	135

WELCOME TO THE PROGRAM

Take a deep breath. Put a smile on your face, and tell yourself, "This is going to be the beginning of the end."

Feel relieved? You should.

No doubt you have made a few, or more than a few, attempts to lose weight before. A stack of diet books on the kitchen counter or an attractive sweat suit tucked in your closet may be symbols of your efforts. No matter what you tried in the past, the fact remains the same. Something didn't work, and you're ready to start again.

The *Y's Way to Weight Management* is set up so once you make a commitment to begin, each step forward brings you closer to taking charge of your weight and your life. You begin to manage what and who will influence your eating. Armed with the know-how, you take the responsibility for adjusting your lifestyle to work for, not against, you.

"Why the Y?" you may ask. The YMCA has a long track record in the area of "wellness." Starting back in London in 1844 and spreading to Montreal and Boston by 1851, YMCAs have been leading the way in fitness and health for over 130 years. In the United States alone, 2,133 branches, units, camps, and centers are bringing people together for very positive results.

The YMCA is able to draw on a successful past. Trained professionals conducting YMCA weight management programs across the country for over 10 years have been helping thousands of people incorporate the principles of exercise, sound nutrition, and positive eating habits into their lifestyles.

Goal of the Program

The *Y's Way to Weight Management* is designed to help you learn how to take charge of your weight and your life. The goal of the program is to help you develop a lifestyle that will lead to weight loss and permanent weight management. The approach is comprehensive. Looking at what you eat is only one aspect. Looking at your eating behaviors and exercise habits are the other two. All three aspects are equally important.

- **Eating behaviors**
- **Exercise habits**
- **Food choices**

The program will concentrate on strengthening the positive habits you already have in these three areas. Instead of trying to unlearn bad habits, you will focus your energy on developing new ones and learning how to reinforce a more positive lifestyle.

How It Works

Each session gives you a chance to **identify** different factors influencing your weight, to **set goals** for either changing or shaping these factors to work in your favor, and to **plan** to make sure that all you want to happen will.

The program does not take a "one size fits all" approach. No two people are alike. Your problem areas may be completely different from the next person's. Strategies and techniques are presented so you develop the skills to take control of your own personal weight management.

You will also receive tools to keep tabs on your progress so your goals and plans won't slip through the cracks from week to week.

The *Y's Way to Weight Management* is designed for the least amount of hassle on your part. Each class and accompanying chapter in your book is structured in such a way as to help you achieve results.

Not a Diet

You must understand that this program is not designed to make you stop eating. It is not a diet, nor is it a quick fix for a complicated problem.

Diets set people up for failure. One can cheat on a diet, go off a diet, or start a diet "tomorrow." There is no failure in our program. The attitude is positive and the structure realistic and flexible.

Thanks to much research in the area of weight management, we now know that the body does not respond well to very low calorie diets or dieting without the advantages of physical activity and changes in eating behaviors. Quick fix successes will lead only to a string of lifelong failures unless a comprehensive approach to weight management is taken.

Building Success Teams

Unless you're a hermit, you can't manage your weight alone. We live in a world of people. People, whether family, friends, co-workers or others you hardly know, influence your weight management efforts. Some do so in a positive way; others seem to make everything a real challenge.

The *Y's Way to Weight Management* takes a group approach. Working in a group gives you an edge on solving difficult problems. You can bounce around ideas, try out strategies, and ask for help when things get tough. When you begin the program, you also begin building a "Success Team," a team of people to support your weight management efforts and help you develop a determined attitude. Members of your group may eventually become part of your Success Team, as will all the people who affect your life—even those who make it a bit challenging at times.

Commitments and Responsibilities

It is up to you to take responsibility for your progress throughout the program. Other people may influence your efforts, but you must be in control.

The program will work for you only if you work with it in making these commitments:

Attend class—Each session is structured in such a way that through group interaction you will become proficient in problem solving and applying appropriate strategies and techniques to your personal situations.

Practice—Once you decide which strategies and techniques might work in your particular situation, give them a try and practice some new changes in your life.

Keep records—It's hard to change unless you know exactly what you are doing in the first place. During the program, you will use the *Y's Way to Weight Management Log* to pinpoint problem areas and monitor your new successes.

Allocate time—Not only does it take time to read your book and attend classes, it takes a few minutes each day to reflect on what you are doing and make plans for the next day.

A small yet important amount of time is required to get you up and moving around. Some call this exercise; others prefer to look at it as movement. Whatever you call it, the *Y's Way to Weight Management* asks for a commitment to do more than you are presently doing in the way of physical activity.

Make weight management a priority—We all have priorities in life, things that are important to us: friendship, honesty, religion, finishing college. These priorities or values help shape our day-to-day goals. Take a few minutes to think and write down what's most important to you.

When you finish, go back and reorder your priorities. Start with what's most important and give it first priority.

My Priorities in Life

Take a close look at your priorities. Did "losing weight" or "my health" or "feeling good" make the list? In order to lose weight and maintain the loss over a lifetime, you must rank weight management among your top priorities. It may shift from time to time, depending upon certain events in your life, but its importance, its value, must remain high.

Goal-Setting

Goals are what answer the question, "Where am I going?" They give purpose to everything you do and move you closer to enjoying your priorities in life.

Short-term goals will be established each week. You are encouraged to be realistic. There is no reason to set yourself up for guilt or failure when you already know a goal is out of your control or too much to tackle at once.

Goals are one way to measure progress. You will discover early that "weight" is only one measure. Changes in eating and exercise habits are another indication of how you are doing.

The Y's Way to Weight Management is not a race. It's OK to work on the same goal week after week until it becomes part of your everyday routine.

The YMCA encourages a slow, steady weight loss between one and two pounds each week. This can be accomplished through a combination of increased physical activity and decreased calorie intake with positive eating behavior changes. The results will be a lifestyle you can live with for a lifetime.

During each session you will have a chance to set one or two goals to work toward during the upcoming week. The strategies and techniques to achieve these goals are built into a step-by-step "Action Plan." Your weekly plan will change from week to week. The plan is your plan, unique to your situation.

Am I Ready?

Now that you know what's in store, are you ready to commit yourself? You're the one moving through the program, not your spouse or doctor. You have to be the one who is willing to give it a go.

Am I ready?

☐ Yes
☐ No

If your answer is no, we hope that when the time is right, you will seek us out. If the answer is yes, the YMCA welcomes you aboard! We are committed to doing all we can to support your weight management efforts. We're glad you're willing to join in this commitment.

Complete the Y's Way to Weight Management Personal Contract to reaffirm your commitment and acknowledge your responsibilities.

Personal Contract

I understand the following:

- Weight management involves lifestyle changes in my eating behaviors, exercise habits, and food choices.
- I am responsible for achieving my own goals.
- If I work to change, the changes will work for me.
- The group offers feedback and positive support.

Furthermore, I accept the following responsibilities:

- To attend weekly classes
- To keep the weight management Log
- To practice new ways to alter my lifestyle in order to achieve my goals
- To communicate openly and honestly as a member of the group

_____   _____
Signature   Date

1: INCREASING YOUR AWARENESS

What did you have for dinner two nights ago? How about for lunch last Saturday? Did you eat anything while watching TV last night?

Hard to remember? It's no wonder. With everyone on the go these days, eating has become routine, almost unconscious. It's hard just finding the time to eat some days, not to mention trying to remember everything you put into your mouth.

The First Step

The first step toward managing your weight is to find out what you are doing now: what you eat, why you eat, and how your lifestyle is affecting your weight. The most effective way to learn this information is to write things down.

For starters, use the 24-Hour Recall form to record everything you had to eat and drink during the past 24 hours.

- Begin with your most recent meal or snack, and think back.
- List everything, even if you had only a taste. Don't forget coffee breaks at your desk or nibbling before supper.
- Try to record the amounts as you remember them.

24-Hour Recall

Time	What did I eat? How much?

Any surprises? Did you have any problems remembering what you ate? It's not easy relying on memory alone to recall what you are eating.

Keeping track of snacks and nibbling is an eye-opener. It's natural not to count a few bites of cookie dough while you're baking or a taste of peanut butter before tightening the jar. Sometimes we tend to see only what we want to see. Serving sizes get distorted; seconds and thirds may even get overlooked.

You may be telling yourself, "But this isn't a typical day." Nonetheless, it gives you an idea of how unconscious eating can become.

You are ready for the second step toward weight management. Pick a snack from your Recall to look at more closely. If by chance you didn't snack yesterday, select a meal.

Look beyond the actual foods you ate to the circumstances surrounding the snack. Answer these questions. If you can't remember, write "don't know" in the answer space.

Your Signals

Where were you when you ate the snack? _____

What was your mood? _____

What time was it? _____

Were you hungry? _____

Who else was with you at the time? _____

Had you preplanned to eat the snack at that specific time? _____

Answers to these questions start zeroing in on the "signals" that lead to eating. Signals in themselves are not bad. The problem arises when any signal gets out of hand, leading to overeating and eventually overweight.

There are many reasons why we eat. Some start as far back as childhood with that first cookie for being good or a lollipop at the doctor's office for bravery. Signals have been piling up ever since.

What you think you are doing and what you are actually doing may be two different things. During this program, you will begin to sift through your signals, pinpointing those that are causing problems. Take a few minutes to complete the Eating and Lifestyle Questionnaire located in Appendix A. Answer what you think you are presently doing.

Focusing on You

The *Y's Way to Weight Management Log* is the perfect tool for learning more about yourself. It gives you a clearer picture of what you're doing now. Your eating behaviors, food choices, and physical activity habits come into focus.

Weight management *Logs* are used for troubleshooting. They pinpoint problem areas and identify when these problems occur. Prepared with this information, you can begin planning how to approach your particular situation. Once you master some of the techniques in the program, the *Logs* will help you see changes and successes. They're a great way to monitor your progress and keep you motivated.

Each category or column represents a different piece of information to be collected. You won't be recording all the information every day. Categories will be added as you move through the program.

The *Y's Way to Weight Management Log*

Time—List the time when eating starts day or night.

Where am I?—List the place where eating: if home, the room (kitchen table, living room couch); and if out, the location (name of the restaurant, friend's house, car on the way home from work, your desk at work).

Who is with me?—Record "alone" or list names of others present. They don't have to be eating.

How am I feeling?—Record your feelings or mood immediately before or during eating. Typical feelings are "rushed," "tired," "bored," "confused," "depressed," "happy," "content," and "sad." If you have no particular feelings, record "none" or "neutral."

Am I hungry?—You are either hungry or not. If hungry, describe in your own words how hungry: "famished," "not very," and so forth.

What am I eating?—List all the foods and beverages you put in your mouth. Record how things are prepared: fried, baked, etc. List any added condiments, gravy, salad dressing, sauces, and so on.

How much?—List the amounts of all items. Choose measures you will be able to duplicate each week. Ounces, servings, cups, or handfuls are examples.

Calories—As part of the program, you will learn more about the relationship between calories found in food and how they affect weight management. Recording the amount of calories found in foods will make you more conscious of the food choices you make. This category will be explained in more detail in chapters 3 and 6.

Food Groups—This is a system to help you plan your food choices. Ways to use the system are presented in chapter 5.

Physical activity—What kinds of movement activities do you do now? Record additional activity beyond your daily routine and the amount of time spent in each. Include walking.

Exercising heart rate—This is a measure used to monitor how hard you are exercising. Instructions for measuring your rate are presented in chapter 4.

Reward—New behaviors and changes need to be reinforced as an incentive to become permanent habits in your lifestyle. Suggestions for ways to reward your accomplishments are presented in chapter 7.

Weight—On the last page of the *Log* is a space to record your weight once a week. Weigh yourself on the same day every week at approximately the same time.

The weight management *Log* is not a test or a confession. You're on the honor system when recording. The more accurate you are, the more successful you will be in planning and implementing changes.

Tips on Keeping the *Log*

- **Carry your *Log* with you.** If you forget it, jot down the information on a slip of paper or paper napkin and transfer it later.
- **Be prompt.** Make entries immediately before eating or just after. Even if you're busy, take a minute to record. Don't wait until the day of class to record a week's worth of eating! An entry is considered a single meal or snack when 15 minutes pass between bites. If nibbling, continue recording all the information until you stop.
- **Be honest.** Record the foods you are actually eating. Don't just record the successful times or what you wished you would have eaten. Even if you "blew it," or feel you are having a bad day, write everything down.
- **Be complete.** Record all that is asked. Each week you will record different pieces of information. To be of value, your *Log* must be accurate and complete.
- **Reflect.** Take a few minutes each night before going to bed to look over the day. Reflect on how you did and what you would do differently the next time.

Sample Daily Log Entry

The sample below gives you an idea of how to complete the *Log* with information for one day's eating behaviors. Try to be as accurate as possible.

Date FRIDAY

Time	Where am I?	Who is with me?	How am I feeling?	Am I hungry?	What am I eating? How much?	Calories	Fruit/Vegetable	Grain	Milk	Meat	Other
6:30 AM.	KITCHEN	ALONE	TIRED	VERY	1/4 SMALL CANTALOUPE, 1 SHREDDED WHEAT BISCUIT, 1/2 BANANA LOW FAT MILK – ABOUT 2/3 C.						
8:30 AM	WORK – CONFERENCE ROOM	MARY, SUE JEAN	OK	NO	2 DOUGHNUTS, COFFEE W/ CREAM, 2 tsp. SUGAR						
10:00 AM	DESK	ALONE	NEUTRAL	NO	COFFEE, CREAM, 2 tsp. SUGAR						
11:30 AM	CAFETERIA	BOB, ALICE	GREAT	YES	CHEF SALAD, TURKEY, SWISS CHEESE, HAM, CUCUMBERS, TOMATO, LETTUCE, MUSH-ROOMS, 3 TBS. FRENCH DRESSING, ROLL – PLAIN (1) LOWFAT MILK – 8 OZ. CARTON						
2:00 PM	DESK	ALONE	ANXIOUS	NO	2 CANDY BARS						
3:00 PM	CONFERENCE ROOM	MARY, SUE JEAN	NEUTRAL	NO	CHOCOLATE BIRTHDAY CAKE – 2 PIECES						
5:30 PM	CAR	ALONE	TIRED	NO	2 HANDFULS PEANUTS – DRY ROASTED						
7:00 PM	DINING ROOM	FAMILY	HAPPY	YES	BAKED HADDOCK – 4 OZ. W/ BREAD CRUMBS & 1 PAT MARGARINE, TARTAR SAUCE – 2 HEAPING TBS. BROCCOLI – 2 STALKS W/ HOLLANDAISE SAUCE, MIXED GREEN SALAD – DIET DRESSING, BROWN RICE – 1 C. W/ MARG-ARINE, WATERMELON – 2" SLICE						
9:00 PM	DEN	CHILDREN	HAPPY	NO	BOWL OF ICE CREAM – 2 LARGE SCOOPS						
					Daily Totals						

Exercising Heart Rate _____
Physical Activity:

Reward? yes _____ no _____   Weight _____

Extra! Extra! Just by keeping the weight management *Log*, you may start to eat less! Recording gives you a few extra seconds to think about what you're doing. At first, you may find it's easier not to eat something than to have to write it down. After a while, you may realize you're not hungry and really don't need the extra food.

Key Points

- The first step towards weight management is knowing what you are doing now: what you eat, why you eat, and how your lifestyle affects your weight.
- By keeping the *Log*, you can pinpoint problem areas, plan changes, and track your progress.
- Signals often trigger eating. Not all signals are bad.

The Week Ahead

During the upcoming week, write in your weight management *Log*. When you eat, record the time of day or night, whether hungry or not, and the type and amount of food and beverages.

Begin walking. Set a time during the day and in the evening. Ask a friend to join you. Keep track of your activity by jotting it down in the *Log*. Start with at least 15 minutes of activity; then work your way up gradually to 20 minutes, 4 days a week.

Take a few minutes at the end of each day to review your day's *Log* and decide how you might do things differently the next time. If you accomplished your plans for the day, make sure to do something nice for yourself. Start thinking of ways to reward yourself that have nothing to do with food. Chapter 7 presents ideas on ways to establish rewards.

Action Plan

Goals

My goals for the week: _____

_____

_____

Goal-Setting

Plans for the week	Went well	Had problems	Keep practicing

Week in Review

At the end of the week, take a few minutes to look over your *Log* and Action Plan. How did you do? Did you accomplish all your plans? Do some still need work?

Based on your accomplishments, check the appropriate column on the Action Plan for all the plans you listed. If your plans went well, put a check in the first column. If you ran into problems, mark the second column and decide how you would do things differently.

Throughout the program, weigh yourself only once—at the end of the week. Record your weight change on the Weight Graph on the inside of the back cover. Total the time you spent exercising on the Exercise Log on the inside of the front cover.

2: MANAGING YOUR EATING TIME

Have you ever raced out the door without breakfast or gulped down lunch? Why? Is "I don't have time" the answer?

When time gets in the way of your weight loss efforts, you have a time management problem. We usually think of time management in the business sense. The same principles can be applied to your personal life, especially to eating. How you space eating throughout the day, what time you eat, and how quickly or slowly you eat all influence weight management.

Time and Weight Management

One of the most obvious yet ignored problems in managing your eating time is skipping meals. Long lapses between eating only distort hunger. You may know the feeling: "I could eat a house, I'm so hungry."

Becoming overly hungry often ends with eating more calories at one meal than would happen if eating were spaced throughout the day. Snacking can also get out of hand. A harmless snack could lead to a binge. All in all, skipping meals more than catches up with you in terms of total calories eaten in a day.

Another area of eating time management relates to the time when you eat. Calories may be burned more efficiently at various times of the day. Although calories are used even when sleeping, those eaten in the morning are more likely to be burned for energy during the day and those eaten late in the evening are more likely to be stored as fat.

Finishing a meal in record time or eating until you can hardly move are both time management problems. It takes the brain about 20 minutes to receive signals that you're full. Rather than recognizing this fact, some people keep eating and eating and eating until they finally get the signal. Persons who zip through the meal feel a little bored and keep eating to pass the time while others catch up.

The First Step

Ironically, the basis for many eating time management problems stems from poor time management. Daily routines may dictate when we eat and how much time we spend. Crowded schedules, conflicting mealtime activities, and little time to get organized create a new set of time management problems related to eating.

How do you spend your days and evenings? Use the Look-at-a-Glance Worksheet to get an idea of how your time is spent.

Look-at-a-Glance Worksheet

- Jot down the kinds of things you normally do during each hour.
- Note the time when you get up and go to bed; the times when you normally eat breakfast, lunch, and dinner; your work schedule and routine activities during the day.
- If activities take more than the hour, draw a continuous line down the page until the activity ends. Be brief in your descriptions.

Time of day	What am I doing?	Meal	Snack	Nibble
5:00 a.m.				
6:00 a.m.				
7:00 a.m.				
8:00 a.m.				
9:00 a.m.				
10:00 a.m.				
11:00 a.m.				
Noon				
1:00 p.m.				
2:00 p.m.				
3:00 p.m.				
4:00 p.m.				
5:00 p.m.				
6:00 p.m.				
7:00 p.m.				
8:00 p.m.				
9:00 p.m.				
10:00 p.m.				
11:00 p.m.				
Midnight				
1:00 a.m.				
2:00 a.m.				
3:00 a.m.				
4:00 a.m.				

Where Eating Fits

Now that you can clearly see your normal routine, you have something with which to compare your eating pattern. Besides eating the three traditional meals—breakfast, lunch, and dinner—look closely at your *Log* to see what other kinds of eating you are doing throughout the day.

Snacks are either planned or unplanned. They could be the size of a meal. Snacks may replace a meal or be in addition. In comparison to constant nibbling, snacks are deliberate and eaten at one time. Nibbling tends to be eating right out of the bag or in front of the refrigerator or tasting food while cooking. Both snacks and nibbling could lead to binge eating if they get out of control.

Go back through your *Log*, marking M (meal), S (snack), or N (nibble) next to each eating episode. When you're finished, make a slash in the appropriate box next to the time when eating occurred on the Look-at-a-Glance Worksheet.

Start analyzing your eating pattern. See how your daily routine influences your eating time.

Eating Time Profile

To get an even clearer picture of the times you are eating, complete the Eating Time Profile.

- Refer to the Look-at-a-Glance Worksheet when completing this graph.
- Record the number of times during the week when eating occurred by filling in the type of eating with either an M, S, or N in the boxes next to the time frame.
- The sample profile indicates constant eating during the evening. This person has a busy work schedule, skips breakfast and most lunches, and gets home from work late.
- Circle the hour when you normally eat breakfast, lunch, and supper. If you are currently skipping any of these meals, still circle a time you could consider eating the meal.
- After completing the profile, go back to see what's happening in your daily routine. Continuous eating could be a sign that you're bored, with little else to do but eat. Check to see if long lapses in eating are followed by continuous snacking or nibbling.

Eating Time Profile

Sample

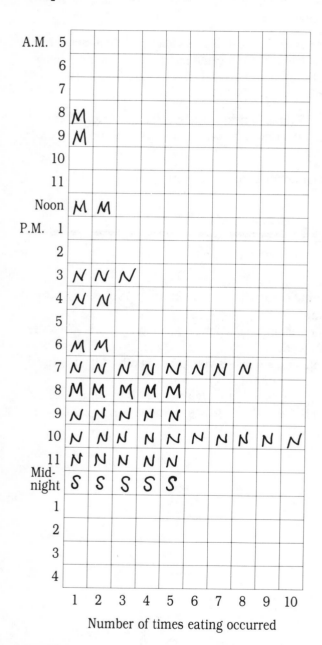

My Eating Time Profile

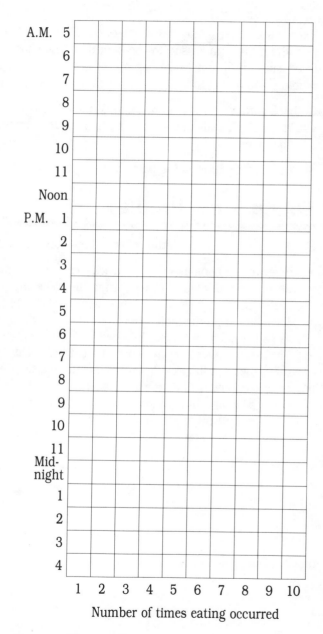

Number of times eating occurred

Adapted from Levitz, L.S., & Jordan, H.A. (1973). Analysis of food intake. *Behavioral Weight Control Program*. Philadelphia: University of Pennsylvania. Copyrighted by and reproduced with permission of Henry A. Jordan, M.D.

Pinpointing Problems

Use the Look-at-a-Glance Worksheet and Eating Time Profile to pinpoint problems in managing your eating time. Make a list of problems you need to work through during the program. Divide them into two areas: **spacing** and **pacing**. Spacing problems tend to deal with skipping meals and sporadic snacking and nibbling. Pacing relates to eating too quickly.

Problem List

Spacing

_____

_____

_____

_____

_____

Pacing

_____

_____

_____

_____

_____

_____

Strategies for Managing Your Eating Time

The following list of strategies offers possible alternatives for solving your problems in managing eating time. Decide which ones are appropriate to try out and practice for your particular situation.

Spacing Eating

If skipping meals is a problem, consider these strategies:

- Space eating throughout the day.
- Use the *Log* to preplan meal times. Jot down the approximate times you are going to eat beforehand.
- Plan to eat at least three times a day.
- Breakfast doesn't have to be at home. Take something to work and eat when you get there or during a planned midmorning break.
- Mark lunch time on your desk calendar.
- Schedule a planned snack during long time lapses.

- Plan a snack as a meal during a time you usually don't eat.
- Divide a large meal into two smaller meals or one small meal and a planned snack. Don't increase your intake; just space it out during the day.

If snacking is a problem, consider these strategies:

- Look at your daily routine. Decide if a snack or break is needed.
- Plan breaks throughout the day to avoid tension buildup. Breaks can be as short as 5 minutes.
- Get up and move around during a break. Stretch, walk, or do another nice thing for yourself.
- Use exercise to unwind.
- Check your daily schedule to see if frequent snacking is related to "down times." Get out of the house and away from food when you have a lot of free time on your hands. Exercise or run errands.
- Decide if hunger or thirst is the problem. Reach for water or a low-calorie, decaffeinated beverage at times other than planned snacks.
- If frequent snacking is a problem, plan no more than two to three snacks a day.
- Meals should be smaller when snacks are planned.
- Snacks and favorite foods do not have to be eliminated entirely. Be reasonable and eat moderately when snacking.
- Plan physical activity before a snack break.
- Set limits on what you will eat. Get foods out, prepare the snack, close and put the containers away, sit down, and enjoy the snack.
- Don't eat at your desk at work; change locations. When eating while working, you're more likely to eat quickly without taking the time to relax and enjoy your food and yourself.
- Close down the kitchen at 8 p.m. Turn off the lights and reroute activities in another direction.

If nibbling is a problem, consider these strategies:

- Turn nibbling into one of your planned snacks.
- Store food out of sight.
- Make sure you're not hungry when you start cooking. Have a light snack before you start.
- Taste food only to season. Use a second spoon to transfer food from the container to a spoon for tasting. Don't taste directly from the container.
- To avoid continuous nibbling while cooking, chew gum or keep a toothpick in your mouth.
- Put ingredients away after you use them.
- When preparing large quantities of food, portion excess into containers and store.
- Avoid the kitchen as much as possible. When waiting for something to finish cooking, leave the room or find another nonfood activity to occupy your time.
- Have other family members make their own snacks and lunches.
- Send leftovers home with guests after a party.

Pacing Eating

If eating quickly is a problem, consider these strategies:

- Introduce a delay at some point in the meal.
- Start a delay with a 30-second pause, and work up to a 2-minute delay.
- Take a brief pause in between two parts of a meal. Put down silverware, sip a beverage, share an anecdote about your day, relax, and then go on eating.
- Take smaller bites. Become more conscious of how volume feels in your mouth. If your cheeks are bulging or it's hard to get more food on the fork, your bites are too large.
- Pause after each bite. Finish one mouthful before taking another. Try putting down silverware or sandwiches between bites. Wait until you swallow, then take another bite.
- Cut foods into small pieces. A hamburger takes longer to eat if it's cut in half.
- Alternate sips of water, coffee, or tea with bites of food. The food will last longer, and the fluid will make you feel full.
- Don't rush through the meal to get to favorite foods. Eat some favorites first.

Key Points

- Analyzing when you eat may show patterns in your eating habits.
- How you plan your day may be contributing to some of your problems in managing eating time.
- Rearranging eating times and slowing down how fast you eat may lead to weight loss.

The Week Ahead

Set some realistic goals related to managing your eating time for you to work toward during the week. Continue the physical activity you started last week. This week add extra steps to your everyday routine.

Record the same information in your weight management *Log*. In addition, compute the number of calories you're eating. Refer to the Calorie Charts located in Appendices E and F. It is important to be as accurate as possible when recording the amount of food you're eating. Accuracy will help you calculate the correct number of calories. Nutrition labels on food packages also tell the amount of calories in a food. Check them out.

Calculating calories takes time. Plan to devote an extra 15 minutes each night to recording and totaling your calories for the day.

Try spacing your eating throughout the day. Jot down the times you want to eat ahead of time in your *Log*.

Select two or three strategies for managing your eating time to try out and practice throughout the week.

Action Plan

Goals

My goals for the week: _____

_____

_____

Goal-Setting

Plans for the week	Went well	Had problems	Keep practicing

Week in Review

At the end of the week, take a few minutes to look over your *Log* to see what changes you made related to spacing eating throughout the day and slowing down your eating pace. Do some still need work?

Based on your accomplishments, check the appropriate column on the Action Plan for all the plans you listed. If your plans went well, put a check in the first column. If you ran into problems, mark the second column and decide how you would do things differently. This may mean trying a different strategy or technique. Even if a technique worked well, you may want to continue working on it. Add any plans you need to carry over on your next week's Action Plan.

How do you feel now that you have started to exercise? Total the time you spent exercising on the Exercise Log on the inside of your book's front cover. Record your weight change on the Weight Graph on the back inside cover.

How did changes in managing eating time influence your eating pattern? Complete an Eating Time Profile for your past week and compare it with the one you completed the week before.

Eating Time Profile

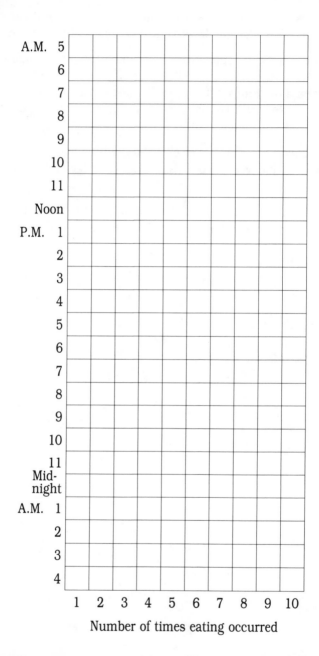

Number of times eating occurred

3: CALCULATING ENERGY COSTS

Calories. Just the sound of the word is enough to make some people cringe. To the seasoned dieter calories are taboo, almost sinful. This is unfortunate because we all need calories to live.

There is nothing wrong or bad about calories. The problem in weight management occurs when the number of calories eaten is more than what the body uses every day. Or stated another way, the problem occurs when physical activity is too low for the amount of calories consumed. Compounding the problem are the low calorie diets claiming an easy and fast way to "drop pounds."

What is a Calorie?

A calorie is a unit of measurement. Think of it as you do other measurements—inches to measure distance or grams to measure weight. The calorie (abbreviated "kcal") is used to measure the amount of energy in foods and beverages. This energy goes to work keeping our bodies functioning and moving us along when we're active. We even need energy when we're sleeping or sitting quietly just thinking. When food is metabolized in our bodies, it releases energy and heat that can be measured in calories. Our bodies use energy to keep us alive and functioning.

Nutrients and Calories

Foods are made up of nutrients. There are six major nutrient categories.

1. Protein
2. Carbohydrate
3. Fat
4. Vitamin
5. Mineral
6. Water

The first three—protein, carbohydrate, and fat—are the ones supplying energy. Contrary to many advertising claims and testimonials, vitamins and minerals will not give you pep and energy. They do not contain calories, though they are essential in making your body function properly. In addition to the first three nutrients, alcohol (a non-nutrient) also supplies calories. There are 7 calories per gram (kcal/g) of alcohol, almost as much as fat.

Carbohydrate—provides energy at 4 kcal/g
Protein—provides energy at 4 kcal/g
Fat—provides energy at 9 kcal/g

The amount of carbohydrate, protein, and fat in a food determines the caloric value of that food. Each food varies in the amount of any of these three nutrients. Foods like meat, fish, and poultry contain protein and fat and no carbohydrate, while fruits are mostly carbohydrate.

By using information on food labels, you can calculate the source of your calories. Most calorie figures are rounded off for the label. The figure usually seen on a carton of whole milk is rounded off to 150 calories. For example, by reading the nutrition label on a milk carton, you know an 8-ounce glass of milk has the following:

8 g of fat
8 g of protein
11 g of carbohydrate

To determine the amount of calories each nutrient contributes to milk, multiply the number of grams by the calories per gram:

$$8 \text{ g fat} \times 9 \text{ kcal} = 72 \text{ kcal}$$
$$8 \text{ g protein} \times 4 \text{ kcal} = 32 \text{ kcal}$$
$$\underline{11 \text{ g carbohydrate} \times 4 \text{ kcal} = 44 \text{ kcal}}$$
$$\text{Total Calories} = 148 \text{ kcal for 8 oz}$$

After you calculate the source of calories, it's obvious that most of the calories in milk come from fat. This is one reason why lowfat milk, with only 2 grams of fat, or skim milk, with none, is more appealing in a weight management program.

Knowing how to calculate the amount of calories will give you a clear picture of where your calories are coming from.

Too Much of a Good Thing

Weight management becomes an issue when an overabundance of calories has to go somewhere. That "somewhere" is storage—in the form of fat. All excess calories not used by the body are converted to fat. It doesn't matter whether the calories come from extra carbohydrate, protein, or fat.

It takes an excess of 3,500 calories to create a pound of body fat. You see this as another pound on the scale. Most people can't believe it takes 3,500 calories to gain a pound. Believe it—it's true. Of course, the buildup doesn't happen overnight. Weight gain seems to creep up each year.

Moving Fat Out of Storage

Knowing that excess body fat is stored energy should make you realize that "storage" is another place where the body can get calories for things it needs to do. Moving fat out of storage, using it, and preventing future calories from being put into storage is what weight management is all about.

The *Y's Way to Weight Management* emphasizes reducing the amount of stored fat in your body as one goal in the program. Your percent body fat was measured during the preassessment and will be used to gauge your progress in reducing stored fat.

The YMCA fitness programs use 16% body fat for men and 23% for women as desirable measurements. Based on where you were at the beginning of the program, goals were established to help you work toward these figures.

How Many Calories You Need

The number of calories you need depends upon the number of calories you use in a 24-hour period. Think of this number as your "Total Energy Cost." Once you determine your Total Energy Cost, you can compare it with the number of calories you are actually eating. If the two figures aren't close, it's likely you have a weight management problem. If the figures are close, you may be maintaining too high a weight and still need to make changes. The next step is to develop a sound plan to boost your Total Energy Cost and lower your caloric intake.

Total Energy Cost

There are three "costs" or ways your body uses energy. The sum of these costs makes up your Total Energy Cost.

1. **Living Cost** is the energy used just for living. This is referred to as your basal metabolic rate (BMR). It includes calories needed to breathe, make your heart beat, and carry out other essential functions.
2. **Activity Cost** is the energy needed for everything you do during the day. This cost may be calculated using a factor representing your activity level. Other methods for determining this cost involve detailed calculations for activities performed during each hour of the day.
3. **Eating Cost** is also referred to as the specific dynamic action of food. It represents the energy used just to digest food. Ironically, this cost is very minor.

Complete the three energy cost worksheets to determine each of your costs. Compute your Total Energy Cost by adding all three costs together in Worksheet 4.

The worksheet formulas let you calculate your estimated calorie needs. Remember they are only an estimate. Your past dieting habits, amount and frequency of exercise, as well as other factors that are difficult to control with formulas affect the final figures.

When completing the worksheets, keep these points in mind:

- As you get older, your basal metabolic rate drops. Your body doesn't need as many calories to keep going. If you are eating the same amount of food as you did when you were 25 and you're now 45, you are likely to gain weight.
- Men usually have a higher basal metabolic rate than women. This may be true for a number of reasons. They often have more lean tissue (muscle). Muscle has a higher metabolic rate than fat. Also, their body surface area may be larger.
- As you will read shortly, your past dieting efforts may affect your present basal metabolic rate. This figure may actually be lower than calculated.

Worksheet 1: Calculating Your Living Cost

Step 1. On the surface area chart below, put a dot at your height on the left scale and another dot at your current weight on the far right scale.

Step 2. Using a straight edge, draw a line to connect both dots. The point at which the line crosses the middle scale is your surface area. (In the example shown, surface area is 1.49.)

Step 3. Locate the number of calories per surface area for your age and sex on the "Calorie/Surface Area" chart.

Step 4. Multiply Step 2 by Step 3.

_____
Surface Area

_____
Calorie/Surface Area

_____
Living Cost

Chart for Determining Surface Area

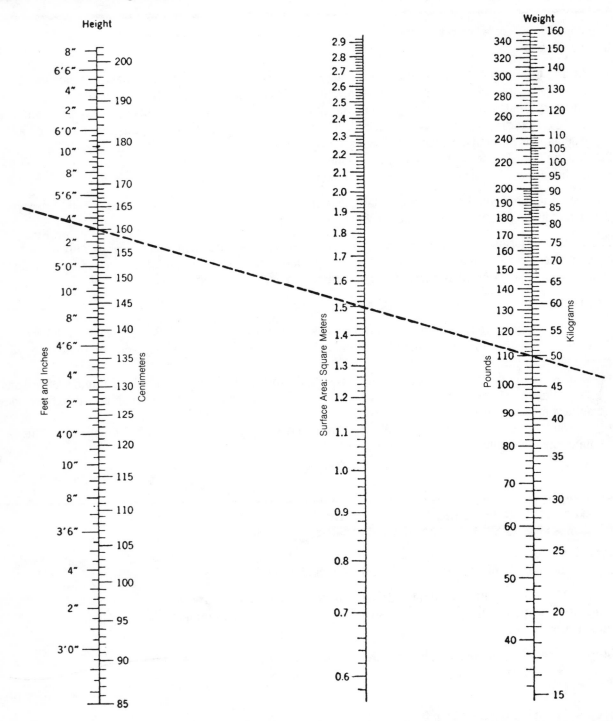

Height

Weight

Surface Area: Square Meters

Note. From W.M. Boothby, J. Berkson, & H.L. Dunn. (1936). "Studies of the energy metabolism of normal individuals: A standard for basal metabolism, with a nomogram for clinical applications. *American Journal of Physiology,* **116**, 468-484. Reprinted by permission.

Calorie/Surface Area/24 Hours

Age (yr)	Men	Women
20-24	941	845
25-29	912	840
30-34	894	839
35-39	882	830
40-44	876	823
45-49	871	814
50-54	864	802
55-59	850	790
60-64	835	778
65-69	816	763
70-74	794	751
75	763	746

Note. Values are smoothed means of basal calories per square meter for 24 hours from the three largest and most authoritative sets of standards. The Mayo Foundation Standards of Boothby, Berkson, and Dunn, based on measurements of 639 males and 828 females; the British measurements of Robertson and Reid, 987 males and 1,323 females; and The Carnegie Nutrition Laboratory data of Harris and Benedict, 136 males and 103 females. Adapted from "Metabolism." In *Biology Data Book*, pp. 1529-1530. Edited by Philip L. Altman and Dorothy S. Dittmer. Bethesda, MD: Federation of American Societies for Experimental Biology, 1974.

Worksheet 2: Calculating Your Activity Cost

Step 1. Insert the Living Cost figure from Worksheet 1.

_____
Living Cost

Step 2. Determine your activity factor from the activity descriptions below. (When selecting your activity factor, be careful not to overestimate your level of activity. It is better to select the category *below* your estimated activity.)

_____
Activity Factor

Step 3. Multiply Step 1 by Step 2.

_____
Activity Cost

Daily Activity Factors[1]

Read each activity description. Pick the one that best describes how you spend your day.

Activity Factor ".1"—You do little more than lie in bed. You may take short walks to the kitchen or bathroom. You tend to spend most of your day in bed.

Activity Factor ".2"—You tend to spend most of your time in bed or in a chair. You may walk around the house from room to room or watch a little television.

Activity Factor ".3"—You expend your energy doing light housework, minor chores, or errands. There is no sweat involved in your activity, which might be anything from casually vacuuming the carpet to bird watching.

Activity Factor ".4"—You probably have a steady job. Perhaps you work in an office and spend your energy by sitting at a desk all day. Maybe your job entails typing or walking from floor to floor (climbing a few stairs in the process). At nighttime, your activity is low. Perhaps you watch television or read a good book. However, you probably spend a calm, low-energy, relaxing evening at home.

Activity Factor ".5"—You have a steady job that requires climbing stairs, extensive walking, etc. Your day is usually busy and hectic, and when you finally arrive home, you probably mow your lawn or do some gardening. Perhaps this is your night to play racquetball, go to the spa, or take care of young, active children. You often feel small bursts of energy and therefore follow an inconsistent exercise pattern. The work you do, however, possibly causes you to perspire and results in a fair amount of energy expenditure.

Activity Factor ".6"—You have a job but also welcome some sort of daily physical exercise. Perhaps you run 6 miles a day before you go to work. Maybe after work you swim a few laps. Perhaps you attend dance class for 1½ hours. Your activity is consistent.

Activity Factor ".7"—You perform light manual labor, something to build up sweat and strain. You don't lift a 20-lb sledgehammer all day; however, you are probably exposed to the sun or working under strained conditions. When you come home, you pursue some form of exercise.

Activity Factor ".8"—You are most likely performing hard manual labor daily. You are one of those people who does lift a 20-lb sledgehammer all day. You work hard and long, and you exercise hard as well. Your muscles are well toned, and you are used to everyday exhilaration.

Activity Factor ".9"—You exercise almost continuously and your body is almost always in constant motion.

Activity Factor "1"—You are probably a conditioned athlete, training for a marathon or perhaps even the Olympics. You are in top physical condition and you do extensive, efficient training daily.

[1]From *The Complete Diet Workbook* (pp. 43-43) by W.P. Steffee, 1982, Norwalk, CT: Appleton-Century-Crofts. Adapted by permission.

Worksheet 3: Calculating Your Eating Cost

Step 1. Insert the Living Cost figure from Worksheet 1.

_____
Living Cost

Step 2. Insert the Activity Cost figure from Worksheet 2.

_____
Activity Cost

Step 3. Add Steps 1 and 2.

_____

Step 4. Multiply Step 3 by ".06".

_____
Eating Cost

Worksheet 4: Calculating Total Energy Cost

Step 1. Insert the Living Cost figure from Worksheet 1.

_____
Living Cost

Step 2. Insert the Activity Cost figure from Worksheet 2.

_____
Activity Cost

Step 3. Insert the Eating Cost figure from Worksheet 3.

_____
Eating Cost

Step 4. Add Steps 1, 2, and 3 for your Total Energy Cost.

_____
Total Energy Cost

As you begin to increase your exercise, a shift in your activity cost will keep your total energy cost up. Although your living cost will decrease as your weight drops, the drop will be less significant if exercise is increased. In fact, your basal metabolic rate will actually increase when you exercise. You will read more about this shortly.

Where You Stand

Select three normal days in your _Log._ Total the number of calories eaten each day. Divide this figure by three to determine the average number of calories you consume in a day. The Calorie Charts located in Appendices E and F will help you compute the number of calories in the foods you ate. Remember that this figure is an estimate.

Average caloric intake: _____

How does the number of calories you ate compare with your Total Energy Cost? If your caloric intake is lower, you may have already started cutting back on total calories and increasing physical activity. That's terrific! In order to lose weight, an upset must take place in the balance of energy you consume and use. This is referred to as "unbalancing the energy equation."

Unbalancing the Energy Equation

One of the goals in weight management is to keep the total energy cost up as a result of increasing physical activity while gradually lowering the calories you eat. This helps your body use the calories you are eating as well as the stored calories (fat) you have accumulated. By doing this, you avoid having "leftover" calories. You can think of this goal as _unbalancing the energy equation._

There are three main equations related to weight management. When your weight is stable, the energy equation is balanced, which means the calories you eat are equal to or close to the calories you use for your Total Energy Cost. The **balanced equation** looks like this:

Energy in = Energy used

A shift in this equation can lead either to weight gain or to weight loss as shown in the following two equations.

Weight gain—Taking in more calories than you use causes a shift in the equation. Excess calories are deposited as fat, and weight is gained:

$$\text{Energy in} > \text{Energy used}$$

Weight loss—To unbalance the equation in favor of losing weight, the total number of calories eaten must decrease *and* the number of calories used must increase. This increase in calories used occurs by increasing physical activity:

$$\text{Energy in} < \text{Energy used}$$

Dieting—*Not* the Answer

As the explanation for the weight loss equation explains, losing weight involves a combination of eating fewer calories *and* increasing the amount of calories used each day. Dieting without increasing physical activity will only work *against* your weight management efforts.

Dieting alone tends to lower the body's living cost or basal metabolic rate (BMR). This means your body actually slows down and uses fewer calories just to live. On severely restrictive diets, this decrease in your BMR can be as high as 45%! In the case of dieting, the less you eat, the slower your body works and the (relatively) less weight you lose than if you were more active while dieting.

With many repeated dieting attempts, the body begins to adjust to lower and lower resting metabolic rates after each try. The vicious circle of repeated dieting causes the body to conserve energy. This makes dieting progressively less effective. Plateaus start to occur, and weight losses become less than you would expect.

In addition to a lower basal metabolic rate, a significant amount of lean tissue or muscle is lost when dieting. The benefits of combining exercise with a mild calorie restriction include losing primarily fat, not muscle. Muscles are also toned with exercise so you start to look more fit.

The Importance of Increasing Exercise

Incorporating exercise into your weight management adds benefits you probably never dreamed of. If there ever was a secret to losing weight, consider it exercise.

Exercise helps your body burn *more* calories than you would dieting alone. It does this by raising the basal metabolic rate so you continue to burn calories long *after* you *stop* the activity. The basal metabolic rate can rise as much as 7 to 28% up to 4 to 6 hours after exercise. If your BMR is 1,870 calories, this could mean 131 to 524 additional calories used just because you suited up and exercised! Don't forget you also benefit from the calories used during the activity itself.

Some people fear the benefits of exercise will be offset by increasing their appetite. They picture themselves eating back all these used calories. That is simply not true. Exercise up to an hour actually *decreases* the appetite. Any slight increases in appetite after exercising strenuously for a very long time, beyond an hour, are compensated by the increases in calories burned during the exercise session. Exercise also gets you away from food. You can't be putting on weight if you're out exercising.

One of the most valuable benefits from exercise is how it makes you feel. Ask anyone who's hooked on exercise. You start to feel good about yourself and about what you're doing for your body. Exercise is also a great technique to reduce stress. All in all, exercise works for you, not against you.

How to ''Do It'' to ''Lose It''

The rate at which you decide to lose weight will determine how many fewer calories to eat and how much more activity to incorporate into your schedule. Sound and effective weight loss is at a rate between 1 to 2 pounds per week. Use the following guide to determine your daily caloric deficit. For example, if you want to lose 1 pound a week, a 500-calorie deficit each day must be made. This can be achieved by eating fewer calories and increasing exercise. This deficit adds up to 3,500 calories at the end of a week (500 kcal × 7 days = 3,500 kcal). Remember, it takes 3,500 calories either to lose or to gain a pound.

Desired rate of weight loss per week	Caloric deficit per day
½ lb	250 kcal
1 lb	500 kcal
1½ lb	750 kcal
2 lb	1,000 kcal

Combining one of the caloric deficit figures with four weekly exercise sessions that use up 200 calories per session is a realistic goal when starting a weight management program. Once this goal is reached, expand it by increasing the calories used during a workout.

The estimated number of calories used for a particular activity is based on a person's weight. A heavier person will burn more calories than a lighter person doing the same activity for a similar length of time. This definitely is *not* meant to be an incentive to weigh more. It means that the body has to exert more energy to move the greater body mass of the heavier person.

The Activity Chart lists the amount of time required to burn 100 calories in a particular activity. Use this information to plan an exercise program that will support your weight loss efforts. The amount of time in an activity is computed for different weights. Select the weight level closest to your own. For example, if you weigh 150 pounds, you would have to walk approximately 36 minutes to use 200 calories.

Activity Chart

Activity	Weight (kg) (lb)	Time (min) to use 100 kcal based on body weight						
		55 / 120	59 / 130	68 / 150	77 / 170	86 / 190	96 / 210	105 / 230
Aerobic dance[a]		22	20	18	16	14	13	11
Badminton		19	17	15	13	12	11	10
Basketball		13	12	11	9	8	8	7
Canoeing		41	39	33	30	26	24	22
Climbing (no pack)		15	14	12	11	10	9	8
Backpacking (10 lb pack)		14	13	11	10	9	8	7
Cycling (5.5 mph)		28	26	23	20	18	16	15
Stationary biking		17	15	13	12	11	9	9
Ballroom dancing		36	33	29	25	23	20	19
Fast dancing		11	10	9	8	7	6	6
Gardening (digging)		14	13	12	10	9	8	8
Mowing		16	15	13	12	10	9	9
Raking		34	31	27	24	22	19	18
Golf		21	20	17	15	14	12	11
Handball		9	8	7	6	5	5	4
Horseback riding		24	23	20	17	16	14	13
Racketball		9	8	7	6	5	5	4
Running, 11½ min/mi		13	13	11	10	9	8	7
Running, 9 min/mi		9	9	8	7	6	5	5
Walk jog, 13½ min/mi		18	17	15	13	12	10	10
Cross country skiing[b]		13	12	10	9	8	7	7
Skiing, soft snow[c]		17	16	14	12	11	10	9
Squash		9	8	7	6	5	5	4
Swimming, backstroke		11	10	9	8	7	6	6
Swimming, breast stroke		11	10	9	8	7	6	6
Swimming, slow crawl		14	13	11	10	9	8	7
Table tennis		27	25	22	19	17	15	14
Tennis		17	16	13	12	11	10	9
Volleyball		36	34	29	26	23	21	19
Walking, asphalt surface		23	21	18	16	15	13	12

[a]Calculations for aerobic dance are based on averaging the energy expenditure used during the total activity time including stretching, calisthenics, warm-up and cool-down exercises, and actual dance.

[b]Calculations are based on values for skiing, hard snow, level, walking.

[c]Calculations are based on an average of figures for men and women.

Putting It All Together

Use the Energy Rx for Weight Loss worksheet to develop a plan to increase your physical activity and decrease caloric intake. When setting your goals, refer back to the Activity Chart and to measurements taken during the preprogram assessment and recorded on your Weight Profile.

Energy Rx for Weight Loss

Target weight _____ pounds based on _____ % fat

Weight loss rate _____ pounds per week

Number of weeks to reach target weight _____

Intermediate goals _____

_____

Calorie deficit _____ per day

Changes I Am Going to Make to Meet My Calorie Deficit

Physical Activity

Use _____ calories in exercise _____ days a week.

Select activities from the Activity Chart based on your current weight.

Activities	Length of time
_____	_____
_____	_____
_____	_____
_____	_____
_____	_____
_____	_____

Extra steps I can add to my routine to use more calories.

_____

_____

Eating Behavior and Food Choices

Eat _____ fewer calories per day.

List ways to cut down on total calories. Include changes in eating behaviors and food choices (i.e., switch to lowfat milk, half portions, special dessert only once a week).

Foods/behaviors	Estimated calorie savings

Key Points

- Calories are a measure for the potential energy in a food.
- Excesses in total calories are converted to fat and stored in the body.
- Protein, carbohydrate, fat, and alcohol supply calories.
- The total number of calories used by the body in a day is the sum of calories used to live (basal metabolic rate), calories used during activity, and energy used to digest food.
- As people grow older, a drop in physical activity and a decrease in basal metabolic rate contribute to weight gain.
- Decreasing caloric intake and increasing physical activity, in combination, will effectively unbalance the energy equation for weight loss.

The Week Ahead

Plan your physical activity goals to use up an additional 200 calories 4 days a week. Continue recording the time of day, whether hungry or not, and the kind and amount of food you're eating as well as your physical activity. Set aside about 15 minutes each night to record the number of calories you ate. Use the Calorie Charts found in Appendices E and F and food labels to estimate caloric values. Begin pinpointing excess calories, and start cutting back on your total caloric intake.

Action Plan

Goals

My goals for the week: _____

_____

_____

Goal-Setting

Plans for the week	Went well	Had problems	Keep practicing

Week in Review

At the end of the week, take a few minutes to look over your *Log* and Action Plan. How did you do? Did you accomplish all your plans? Do some still need work?

Based on your accomplishments, check the appropriate column on the Action Plan for all the plans you listed. If your plans went well, put a check in the first column. If you ran into problems, mark the second column and decide how you would do things differently. This may mean trying a different strategy or technique. Even if a technique worked well, you may want to continue working on it. Add any plans you need to carry over on your next week's Action Plan.

Record your weight change on the Weight Graph. Total the time you spent exercising and calories used during the activities on the Exercise Log.

4: DEVELOPING AN EXERCISE PLAN

Fitness means different things to different people. To some it may mean being free from aches and pains and having the flexibility to bend and stretch. To others it means having enough energy to play with the kids after a hard day at the office. Whatever the definition, fitness means being able to say, "I feel great!"

Fitness in the broad sense includes physical, mental, emotional, social, medical, and nutritional fitness. Physical fitness is the part of total fitness that deals with the effects of exercise on the body. Becoming fit is more than getting in shape. It's a combination of developing the following:

- Cardiovascular fitness
- Muscle strength and endurance
- Flexibility

Cardiovascular fitness, sometimes called endurance or stamina, refers to the heart's ability to pump blood and the blood vessels' ability to carry blood to the muscle cells in order to process oxygen and carry away waste products. Because oxygen is used during endurance type activity, cardiovascular fitness is also referred to as "aerobic."

Changes in your heart, blood vessels, and lungs take place when you start incorporating endurance type activity in your exercise plan. Your heart is a muscle, and just like other muscles, it will increase in size and weight during an exercise program for fitness. The blood vessels surrounding the heart will branch out further, offering more routes for blood to travel. The lungs, where the blood picks up the oxygen, become more efficient. As a result, your heart becomes stronger, pumping more blood more efficiently with each beat. You end up pumping more blood with fewer beats per minute.

Muscular strength is the ability of a muscle to exert force and overcome resistance. **Muscle endurance** is the ability of the muscles or groups of muscles to persist, to keep going in an activity or movement. Put simply, with adequate strength you can perform an activity for a short time, but muscle endurance lets you continue longer. Muscular strength is needed to stand up; muscular endurance is what keeps you standing for a while.

Flexibility is the ability to use a muscle throughout its full range of motion. In other words, flexibility is the ability to move your joints, to bend, stretch, and twist them easily. Maintaining good joint movement reduces the risk of injury and soreness.

Exercise—The Plus in Your Life

If the benefits from exercise for weight management weren't enough to convince you of its merits, here are some pluses it brings to your total health.

+ Helps decrease the amount of fat deposited in blood vessels.
+ Strengthens bones. The pushing and pulling on bones that goes along with exercise leads to denser, stronger bones.
+ Improves the ability to fall asleep quickly and sleep well.
+ Tones muscles.

+ Helps in coping with stress.
+ Provides fitness benefits including cardiovascular conditioning, muscular strength, and flexibility.

Regular exercise even makes exercising itself more enjoyable. You will be able to exercise longer before getting tired, and recovery after an exercise workout is faster. Most importantly, exercising and becoming fit help you feel good about yourself and improve your outlook on life.

Not all activities provide the same fitness benefits. Some are better for cardiovascular conditioning; others add muscular strength and flexibility. Compare your favorite activities with their fitness benefits listed on the Activity and Fitness Benefits Chart located in Appendix B.

Choosing an Activity

When choosing activities to incorporate in your exercise plan, be sensible. Consider these five traits when evaluating your choices. After listing and evaluating your favorite activities, select one or two to try out during the next week. Select those that offer the greatest number of pluses. For example, choose something

- you enjoy,
- you are able to do for a lifetime,
- compatible with your lifestyle,
- readily available, and
- leading to weight loss and cardiovascular fitness.

My Favorite Activities

List all the activities you enjoy. Place a plus (+) in the appropriate box under each trait.

Activity	Enjoyable	Lifelong	Compatible	Available	Fitness

A Plan That Works

In order to get the most out of an exercise program for both fitness and weight management, the activities you choose must be done frequently for a minimum amount of time each session and should be hard enough to have an effect on your cardiovascular system. An effective exercise plan has these three elements:

1. Frequency
2. Duration
3. Intensity

Frequency—When starting a weight loss program, build in an activity session 4 days a week.

Duration—In order to see improvement in cardiovascular fitness and fat loss, movement must keep up for 20 to 30 minutes.

Intensity—To improve cardiovascular fitness, you must work up a certain heart rate while exercising. This rate is referred to as your *target heart rate*. The safe range for a target heart rate is 60 to 80% of one's maximum heart rate. When beginning an exercise program, it's important to start slowly, exercising at the low end of your target heart rate—around 60%.

In addition to determining your exercising heart rate, another guideline is used to monitor how hard you are working. This is referred to as your rate of perceived exertion. This rate deals with how you feel while exercising. An excellent way to gauge your effort is to be able to talk while you exercise. If you can't carry on a conversation without gasping for breath, slow down.

Take a few minutes to determine your target heart rate and measure your exercising heart (pulse) rate.

Worksheet 1: Determining Your Target Heart Rate

Step 1. Subtract your age (in years) from 220 to find your predicted maximum heart rate (MHR):

220 – _____ = _____
      (age)

(Maximum Heart Rate)

Step 2. Multiply Step 1 by .60 to determine your target heart rate for starting a fitness program.

Target Heart Rate
(60% MHR)

Worksheet 2: Monitoring Your Exercising Heart Rate

Step 1. Insert your exercising heart (pulse) rate. (Within 15 seconds after ceasing exercise, determine your pulse rate. Place your right index finger and middle finger on the left side of your left wrist along the tendons just below the base of your thumb. With a watch, count the pulse beats that you feel for 10 seconds and multiply that number by six.)

_____
(Exercising Heart Rate)

Step 2. Compare your target heart rate from Worksheet 1 with your exercising heart rate.

Starting Up

Start an exercise program sensibly. Include warm-up and cool-down exercises along with your activity period. If you are 35 or older, the YMCA recommends a physical and fitness evaluation before starting an exercise program.

Warm-up—Before starting your activity, spend at least 5 to 10 minutes stretching, bending, and loosening up. This is a good time to include strength and muscle endurance exercises. Besides improving flexibility, the warm-up gradually increases the activity of the heart and circulatory system.

Activity period—Select aerobic exercises from among your list of favorites. Continue exercising for 20 to 30 minutes. When starting an exercise program for the first time, begin slowly and pace yourself. Try your activity for 10 to 15 minutes the first week, and work up from there.

Cool-down—Consider this recovery time. Incorporate 5 to 10 minutes of slow movement. This helps blood return to the heart and allows the body temperature to lower gradually. The best time to take your exercising heart rate is within the first 15 seconds following exercise.

Taking Heed

Listen to your body. During exercise certain signals let you know you are overdoing it. Slowing down or stopping when exercise is too strenuous can save you a lot of aches and pains in the long run.

Warning Signals: Slow down and exercise a little less if any of these signals appear.

- Excessive heart rate
- Labored breathing
- Pale skin or flushness

Danger Signs: Although the warning signals do not indicate immediate danger, only a caution to slow down, the danger signs are more serious and warrant stopping immediately.

- Labored breathing (difficult breathing, not the deep breathing normally associated with exercise)
- Loss of coordination
- Dizziness
- Tightness in chest

Exercising Tips

Dress for comfort and the weather.

When it's warm, follow these simple tips:

- Wear as little as possible. Make sure clothing fits loosely.
- On humid days, carry a washcloth and wipe off perspiration. This helps cool you down.
- Exercise during cooler parts of the day, such as early morning or early evening after the sun goes down.
- Drink lots of water. Refer to the eating and exercise tips.
- Pay close attention to warning signals and signs of heat exhaustion.

When it's cold, protect yourself using these tips:

- Wear one layer less of clothing than you would wear if you were outside but not exercising. It's better to wear several layers of clothing than one heavy layer.
- Cover as much of the body as possible. Insulation traps air warmed by the body, holding it near the skin to prevent heat loss.
- Choose fabrics that allow a two-way exchange of air through layers of clothes, prevent overheating and excessive perspiring, and protect the body against chilling.
- Wear loosely fitting clothes.
- Protect yourself with a hat and turtleneck or scarf. Even a towel wrapped around your neck will do in a pinch. Over 40% of body heat is lost through the head and neck.
- Cover your feet and hands. Mittens offer more warmth and protection than gloves.

Shoes are also important:

- Wear properly fitted shoes.
- Athletic stores can help you determine the type of shoe to wear for the activities you choose.

Eating and Exercise

Follow these tips on eating and exercising:

- Drink six to eight glasses of fluids throughout the day.
- Avoid strenuous exercise for at least 2 hours after eating
- If you exercise vigorously, wait about 20 minutes before eating.
- Avoid eating or drinking anything except water before exercising. This includes candy bars and sodas. They can actually make you feel tired or dizzy once you begin exercising.
- Follow up your exercise session with a glass or two of cool water. Pounds lost on the scale immediately after activity are only water losses. Losing water weight and becoming dehydrated are dangerous and are not supporting your efforts to lose fat.

Key Points

- Physical fitness is the part of total fitness that deals with the effects of exercise on the body.
- For physical activity to be effective, one must work to a target heart rate (intensity) for a significant duration (20 to 30 minutes) at a regular frequency (3 to 5 times a week).
- When developing an exercise plan, select activities you enjoy, those that are compatible with your lifestyle and readily available, that lead to cardiovascular fitness and weight loss, and that are likely to be continued for a lifetime.
- Gradual warm-up and cool-down exercises are an important part of a workout.
- Pay attention to early warning signals and danger signs while exercising.

- Dress properly for both warm and cold weather before going out to exercise.
- Wait 2 hours after eating before exercising. Follow up your activity by drinking one to two glasses of water.

The Week Ahead

Continue your exercise efforts. This may be a good week to ask a friend to join you in exercising. Make sure you include warm-up and cool-down exercises as part of your activity time. Immediately following exercise, monitor your pulse and record your exercising heart rate in the *Log*. If your rate is greater than the target you calculated, exercise a little slower the next day. Continue recording the time you eat and if you're hungry, record also the kinds and amounts of food and beverages you're eating.

Action Plan

Goals

My goals for the week: _____

_____

_____

Goal-Setting

Plans for the week	Went well	Had problems	Keep practicing

Week in Review

Did you start up a new activity or rekindle a favorite exercise? Take a few minutes to look over your *Log* and Action Plan. How did you do? Did you accomplish all your plans? Do some still need work? Remember to look to see if you are better managing eating times and eating fewer calories.

Based on your accomplishments, check the appropriate column on the Action Plan for all the plans you listed. Add any plans you need to carry over on your next week's Action Plan.

Record your weight change on the Weight Graph. Total the time you spent exercising and calories used on the Exercise Log.

5: MANAGING FOOD CHOICES

Still looking for the "diet"? As we said in the introduction, the *Y's Way to Weight Management* gives you the tools to make nutritionally sound food choices from a variety of foods including your all-time favorites. The quick fix diet has no place in weight management.

If there is no diet, you may be asking "What should I eat?" The Hassle Free Food Guide tells you the kinds and amounts of foods that make up a nutritious diet. But it lets *you* make choices to fit your eating style and health needs.

The Hassle Free Food Guide was developed by the United States Department of Agriculture. You've probably seen it before, but never thought of it as a guide for weight management. The Food Guide divides commonly eaten foods into five groups according to the nutritional contributions they make. By following the Food Guide, you'll be able to choose foods for their vitamins, minerals, and protein—as well as caloric content.

The suggested number of servings in the Food Guide averages about 1,200 calories, provides adequate protein, and supplies most of the vitamins and minerals adults need daily. This calorie level—1,200—is the level at which most women are able to lose weight. Most men can usually eat as many as 1,600 calories and still lose weight. When reviewing the Food Guide, keep in mind that the calories listed per serving are an average. This figure varies, depending on the actual foods selected.

One of the goals in weight management is to try to adjust your food choices closer to the suggested number of servings in the Food Guide. This is often best achieved by closely evaluating your choices from the Other Category and balancing selections within the first four groups.

Hassle Free Food Guide

Food group	Suggested number of servings (adults)
Fruit and Vegetable Group	4
Grain Group	4
Milk Group	2
Meat Group (lean meat, poultry, fish, and beans)	2
Other Category	—

Fruit and Vegetable Group

4 servings

Average calories: 40 kcal/fruit, 25 kcal/vegetable

Dark green, leafy, or orange vegetables and fruits (apricots, mangoes, cantaloupes, nectarines, yellow peaches, and persimmons) are recommended three or four times weekly for vitamin A.

Citrus fruit (oranges, grapefruits, tangerines, and lemons), melons, berries, and tomatoes are recommended daily for vitamn C. If not overcooked, asparagus, broccoli, brussels sprouts, cabbage, cauliflower, collards, kale, dandelion, mustard and turnip greens, rutabagas, and turnips are also noted for vitamin C.

Major Nutrients:

Vitamin A, vitamin C, and carbohydrate

Fruits and vegetables are also good sources of fiber and potassium. Dark green vegetables and some fruits are also valued for riboflavin, folacin, iron, and magnesium. Certain greens—collards, kale, mustard, turnip, and dandelion—provide some calcium. Nearly all vegetables and fruits are low in fat, and none contain cholesterol.

Serving Size:

Count ½ cup as a serving, or a typical portion: one orange, half a medium grapefruit, ¼ cantaloupe, juice of one lemon, a wedge of lettuce, a bowl of salad, one small potato.

A starchy vegetable serving may be substituted for a serving in the grain group because of its high carbohydrate content: corn, lima beans, green peas, potato, squash (winter, acorn, or butternut), or sweet potato.

Grain Group

4 servings

Average calories: 70 kcal/serving

Select whole grains and enriched or fortified grain products. This group includes all products made with whole grains or enriched flour or meal: bread, biscuits, muffins, waffles, pancakes, cooked or ready-to-eat cereals, cornmeal, flour, grits, macaroni and spaghetti, noodles, rice, rolled oats, barley, and bulgur.

Major Nutrients:

Carbohydrate, iron, thiamin (B_1), and niacin

Whole-grain products contribute magnesium, folacin, and fiber. They also provide a small amount of protein and are a major source of this nutrient in vegetarian diets.

Refined products (enriched or not) may be low in some vitamins and trace minerals, which are partially removed from the whole grain in the milling process and are not added.

Serving Size:

Count as a serving 1 slice of bread; ½ bagel, English muffin, or hamburger bun; ½ cup cooked cereal, grits, rice, or barley; ½ cup cooked pasta (spaghetti, noodles, or macaroni); or 1 ounce ready-to-eat cereal. Read labels for the approximate number of crackers equivalent to 70 calories.

Milk Group

2 servings/adult, 4 servings/teenager, 3 servings/child, 4 servings/pregnant woman, 4 servings/lactating woman

Average calories: 150 kcal/serving (based on whole milk)

Includes milk in any form: whole, skim, lowfat, evaporated, buttermilk, and nonfat dry milk; also yogurt, ice cream, ice milk, and cheese, including cottage cheese.

Major Nutrients:

Calcium, protein, and riboflavin

These foods also contain vitamins A, B_6, and B_{12}. They also provide vitamin D when fortified with this vitamin.

Fortified (with vitamins A and D) lowfat or skim milk products have essentially the same nutrients as whole milk products but fewer calories.

Serving Size:

Count one 8-ounce cup of milk as a serving; 1 cup plain yogurt; 1 ounce cheese; ½ cup ice cream or ¾ cup ice milk; or ½ cup cottage cheese. (Note: The calcium content of these food servings varies.)

Meat Group (lean meat, poultry, fish, and beans)

2 servings (2 to 3 oz/serving)

Average calories: 75 kcal/oz

This group includes beef, veal, lamb, pork, poultry, fish, shellfish, organ meats, dry beans or peas, soybeans, lentils, eggs, and peanut butter. Nuts and seeds are usually in this group, but because of their high calorie count for an equivalent amount of protein, it would be wise to consider them in the Other Category.

Major Nutrients:

Protein, iron, phosphorus, vitamin B_{12}, niacin, thiamin (B_1), and vitamin B_6

It's a good idea to vary your choices among these foods as each has distinct nutritional advantages. For example, red meats and oysters are also good sources of zinc. Liver and egg yolks are valuable sources of vitamin A. Dry beans, dry peas, soybeans, and nuts are worthwhile sources of magnesium. The flesh of fish and poultry is relatively low in calories and saturated fat.

Cholesterol, like vitamin B_{12}, occurs naturally *only* in foods of animal origin. All meats contain cholesterol, which is present in both the lean and fat. The highest concentration is found in organ meats and in egg yolks. Fish and shellfish, except for shrimp, are relatively low in cholesterol. (Dairy products also supply cholesterol.)

Serving Size:

Count 2 to 3 ounces of lean, cooked meat, poultry, or fish without bone as a serving. One egg or ½ to ¾ cup cooked dry beans, dry peas, soybeans, or lentils count as an ounce of meat. Although 2 tablespoons peanut butter are similar in protein value, this amount is twice the number of calories. When choosing peanut butter, cut back on the "other" fat you eat during the day.

Other Category

No serving sizes are defined because a basic number of servings is not suggested for this group.

Included in this category are sweets (candy, cake, cookies, donuts, gum, jams, jellies, pastries, pies, soft drinks, sugars, syrups); alcoholic beverages (beer, wine, liquors, liqueurs); and fats (butter, margarine, oils, salad dressings, shortening, bacon, cream, olives, avocados).

Nutritional Value:

These products, with some exceptions, such as vegetable oil, mainly provide calories. Vegetable oils generally supply vitamin E and essential fatty acids. Unenriched, refined bakery products are included here because, like other foods and beverages in this category, they usually provide relatively low levels of vitamins, minerals, and protein compared with calories.

Combination Foods

For most foods, it's rather obvious in which group they are classified. Some foods can be classified into more than one group. Foods that combine ingredients from two or more food groups are called "combination foods." Unless you are making these foods yourself at home and know the ingredients, it takes some thinking to decide into which groups foods fall. The following chart shows examples of combination foods and into which groups they may be classified. It's important to note that these foods usually contain more than one serving from a group, even though only one "x" is marked in the example.

Sample Combination Foods

Food	Fruit/Vegetable	Grain	Milk	Meat	Other
French toast, pancakes, waffles		X		X	X
Burrito, beef & bean		X		X	X
Chicken chow mein	X			X	
Lasagna	X	X	X	X	X
Macaroni and cheese		X	X		
Pizza, cheese	X	X	X		X
Quiche, plain		X	X	X	X
Tacos, beef or chicken	X	X	X	X	X

Water

An essential nutrient, not very obvious in the Food Guide, is water. The body loses about 11 cups of water a day through sweating and other normal losses. Foods high in water, like fruits, vegetables, and milk, begin to replace these losses. An additional 6 to 8 glasses of fluid need to be consumed each day to make up the balance. Drinking water is a low-calorie and healthy way to meet these needs.

How You Rate

Use your *Log* to see how closely your food choices compare to the suggested number of servings in each of the four groups and the "Other" category. Put an "X" in the appropriate column across from the food item. Some foods may have several Xs in a column, especially if portions were larger than those suggested in the Guide. Several columns will be checked for a combination food. Don't forget to mark "other" when you know fat was added in preparation.

Total the number of Xs for the day at the bottom of each day's record. Compare your number of servings to those suggested in the Food Guide.

Look at your food choices throughout the week and check how they compared on the chart below. In general, how do you rate in each group? List the "other" choices you eat frequently.

How Do You Rate?

Food group	On target	High	Low
Fruit/Vegetable Group			
Grain Group			
Milk Group			
Meat Group			
Other: _____			

Making the Guide Work for You

The Guide gives you the basics. You have to choose foods that meet your special needs and likes. You're better off eating a wide assortment of foods from the first four food groups.

The number of calories in the Guide vary depending upon the different choices made within each group, the size of the serving, and the way foods are prepared. Calories vary among foods within the same food group because foods are grouped according to the equivalent nutrient contributions, not just calorie contribution.

Choices made from the Other Category zoom beyond the 1,200 calorie figure. Included in this category are sweets, alcoholic beverages, and fats. Calories in the Other Category aren't any more fattening than calories from the first four groups. It's just that these foods supply many more calories than vitamins and minerals. You aren't getting your money's worth nutritionally by selecting these foods.

As you've seen before, "fat" calories add up quickly. It's unrealistic to think you'll be able to avoid fat condiments like margarine or oil forever. Try narrowing your "fat" choices to 2 to 3 teaspoons a day. A pat of margarine or butter is equivalent to a teaspoon of oil in calories. If most of your foods are fried, or gravy tops off your meats and casseroles, or creamed dishes are the mainstay in your diet, cutting back on fat will be difficult at first. Calories also add up quickly in commercially prepared foods. These calories usually come from added fat in the ingredients and preparation.

Think before choosing from the Other Category. Make a different change in your food choices each day. The chapter on "Lowering Your Calories" offers additional suggestions on ways to modify your eating for weight management while incorporating healthful food choices found in the Food Guide.

Where Your Favorites Stand

Early on, we said that continuing to include favorite foods in your eating was important. It's also important to consider the preferences of other family members. These foods, especially the tempting ones, will be available and easily accessible to you at home.

On the Favorite Foods chart that follows, write down your very favorite foods. Also list those you know are favorites of individual family members. Check in which groups these foods may be classified, and calculate the calories they provide.

For your own favorites, decide how best to plan them into your food choices. Decide to eat high-calorie favorites less often. Planning a reasonable portion of a favorite food less frequently could save a lot of calories without making you feel totally deprived. When reviewing your *Log*, check to see if other people's high-calorie favorites are creeping into your eating, especially because these are readily available. You may need to work out some reasonable compromises with family members so their favorites don't become your problems. Chapter 7 offers strategies for managing problem eating.

Favorite Foods

		Food group				
Your favorites	Calories	Fruit/Veg.	Grain	Milk	Meat	Other
Family favorites						

Food Groups and Nutrients

The nutrients mentioned in the Food Guide are not exclusive to a group. In general, a particular food group represents the most important sources of those nutrients. Smaller amounts may be contributed by foods from different groups as well. No one group supplies all the nutrients your body needs. Eliminating any one of the first four groups will affect your health.

There are about 50 known nutrients, including water, needed for good health. The recommended amounts of those nutrients known to be essential for human health have been established by the Food and Nutrition Board of the National Academy of Sciences. They are known as the Recommended Dietary Allowances (RDAs) and serve as the basis for the United States Department of Agriculture's nutrition labeling found on most cans and packages.

The Hassle Free Food Guide considers the RDAs in the suggested number of servings for each food group. The Food Guide lets you focus your weight management efforts on *food choices* rather than the tedious task of counting calories. Learning where calories come from is an important eye-opener at first. Your knowledge of calories and physical activity is also an incentive to include exercise in your weight management plans.

The Food Guide also spares you the difficult task of adding up all the individual nutrients in the foods you eat. These tedious calculations, even when done with computers, are confusing and somewhat misleading without adequate interpretation by a trained nutrition professional. If not accompanied with sound nutrition counseling, these calculations, often referred to as a "nutritional analysis," might be misinterpreted as a need for nutritional supplements instead of changes and modifications in food choices.

Nutritional Supplements

Nutritional supplements are not recommended when a variety of food choices are made within the Hassle Free Food Guide. Those individuals with certain known nutrition-related health conditions should remember that individualized nutrition counseling by a registered dietitian and medical supervision are recommended to deal with their special nutritional needs. It is important to note that for healthy people, intakes of nutrients beyond the RDAs will not result in improved health or greater resistance to disease. The Nutrient Chart in Appendix C identifies the major food sources of nutrients, their functions, and symptoms for over-dosed amounts of the nutrient. The idea that if a little is good, more should be better is definitely *not* the case when it comes to nutritional supplements.

Healthy Eating

Many people involved in weight management are also asking, "What should I eat to stay healthy?" Hardly a day goes by without someone trying to answer that question. Newspapers, magazines, books, radio, television, and self-proclaimed nutrition experts give advice on what foods to eat or not to eat. Unfortunately, much of this advice is confusing and misleading.

The "Dietary Guidelines for Americans," based on the *Dietary Goals for the United States* prepared by the Select Committee on Nutrition and Human Needs, United States Senate, in 1977 began answering the question of healthful eating with seven nutrition and health guidelines.

The Dietary Guidelines[1] are presented for those who want to combine lower calorie eating with more healthful food choices. They are not meant to confuse weight loss efforts or create a hassle. The "Guide to Fat in Common Foods" chart located in Appendix D incorporates the guidelines on fat, sodium, and sugar in the Hassle Free Food Guide. The chart is an excellent resource for putting the Dietary Guidelines to work for you. Compare the foods you are eating with those listed in the different categories of the chart. As part of your Action Plan, decide how to make more healthful food choices. The Reference Shelf in Appendix G provides a listing of reliable nutrition references to help answer more of your specific nutrition questions.

The guidelines below are suggested for most Americans. They do not apply to people who need special diets because of diseases or conditions that interfere with normal nutrition. As stated in the introduction, people requiring special dietary instructions should consult their physicians and registered dietitians.

- Eat a variety of foods.
- Maintain ideal weight.
- Avoid too much fat, saturated fat, and cholesterol.
- Eat foods with adequate starch and fiber.
- Avoid too much sugar.
- Avoid too much sodium.
- If you drink alcohol, do so in moderation.

Eat a variety of foods. The Hassle Free Food Guide fits the guideline for variety. The greater the variety, the less likely you are to develop either a deficiency or an excess of any single nutrient. Variety also reduces your likelihood of being exposed to excessive amounts of contaminants in any single food item.

Maintain ideal weight. The *Y's Way to Weight Management* provides the tools and techniques to help you achieve your weight loss goals.

The relationships between obesity and health have been highly publicized. Obesity is associated with high blood pressure, increased levels of blood fats (triglycerides) and cholesterol, and the most common type of diabetes. All of these, in turn, are associated with increased risks of heart attacks and strokes.

Avoid too much fat, saturated fat, and cholesterol. People with high blood cholesterol levels have a greater chance of having a heart attack. Other factors can also increase this risk: high blood pressure and cigarette smoking.

Eating extra saturated fat and cholesterol will increase blood cholesterol levels in most people. However, there are wide variations among people. Heredity and the way each person's body uses cholesterol are important. Some people can consume diets high in saturated fats and cholesterol and still keep normal blood cholesterol levels. Other people, unfortunately, have high blood cholesterol levels even if they eat low-fat, low-cholesterol diets.

The recommendations offered in this guideline are not meant to prohibit the use of any specific food item or to prevent you from eating a variety of foods. For example, eggs and organ meats (such as liver) contain cholesterol, but they also contain many essential vitamins and minerals as well as protein. Such items can be eaten in moderation so long as your overall cholesterol intake is not excessive.

- Choose lean meat, fish, poultry, and dry beans and peas as your protein sources.
- Moderate your use of eggs and organ meats (such as liver).
- Limit your intake of butter, cream, hydrogenated margarines, shortenings, and coconut oil, and foods made from such products.
- Trim excess fat off meats.
- Broil, bake, or boil rather than fry.
- Read labels carefully to determine both amount and types of fat contained in foods.

Eat foods with adequate starch and fiber. Carbohydrate is one of the major sources of energy in the diet. If you limit your fat intake, you are able to increase your calories from carbohydrates.

There are two types of carbohydrate foods, complex and simple. Simple carbohydrates, such as sugars, provide calories but little else in the way of nutrients. Complex carbohydrate foods—beans, peas, nuts, seeds, fruits, vegetables, and whole-grain breads, cereals, and other products—contain many essential nutrients in addition to calories.

Increasing your consumption of certain complex carbohydrates can also help increase dietary fiber. Eating more foods high in fiber tends to reduce the symptoms of chronic constipation, diverticulosis, and some types of "irritable bowel." There is also concern that low fiber diets might increase the risk of developing cancer of the colon.

To make sure you get enough fiber in your diet, you should include complex carbohydrate choices from the Food Guide. There is no reason to add fiber to foods that do not already contain it. Adding a highly concentrated source of fiber like bran to a diet naturally rich in fibrous foods has no added benefit and can actually irritate the intestines.

Avoid too much sugar. The major health hazard from eating too much sugar is tooth decay (dental caries). The risk of caries is not simply a matter of how much sugar you eat. The risk increases the more frequently you eat sugar and sweets, especially if you eat between meals and if you eat foods that stick to the teeth.

Obviously, there is more to healthy teeth than avoiding sugars. Careful dental hygiene and exposure to adequate amounts of fluoride in the water are especially important.

Contrary to widespread opinion, too much sugar in your diet does not seem to cause diabetes. The most common type of diabetes is seen in obese adults, and avoiding sugar, without correcting the obesity, will not solve the problem. There is also no convincing evidence that sugar causes heart attacks or blood vessel diseases.

Estimates indicate that Americans use on the average more than 130 pounds of sugars and sweeteners a year. This means the risk of tooth decay is increased not only by the sugar in the sugar bowl but by other products containing sugars.

To avoid excessive sugars, follow these suggestions:

- Use less of all sugars, including white sugar, brown sugar, raw sugar, honey, and syrups.
- Eat less of food containing these sugars, such as candy, soft drinks, ice cream, cakes, and cookies.
- Select fresh fruits or canned fruits without sugar or with light instead of heavy syrup.
- Read food labels for clues on sugar content. If the names sucrose, glucose, maltose, dextrose, lactose, fructose, or syrups appear first, then there is a large amount of sugar.
- Remember, how often you eat sugar is as important as how much sugar you eat.

Avoid too much sodium. Excessive sodium is a major hazard for persons who have high blood pressure. Not everyone is equally susceptible. In the United States, approximately 17% of adults have high blood pressure. Sodium intake is but one of the factors known to affect blood pressure. Obesity also plays a role. At present, it is difficult to predict just who will develop high blood pressure. Since most Americans eat more sodium than is needed, consider reducing your sodium intake.

To avoid too much sodium, follow these suggestions:

- Learn to enjoy the unsalted flavors of foods.
- Cook with only small amounts of added salt.
- Add little or no salt to food at the table.
- Limit your intake of salty foods, such as potato chips, pretzels, salted nuts and popcorn, condiments (soy sauce, steak sauce, seasoned salts), cheese, pickled foods, and cured meats.

Remember that up to half of sodium intake may be hidden, either as a natural part of the food or, more often, as part of a preservative or flavoring agent that has been added. Baking soda, baking powder, monosodium glutamate (MSG), soft drinks, and even many medications contain sodium.

If you drink alcohol, do so in moderation. Alcoholic beverages tend to be high in calories and low in other nutrients. Even moderate drinkers may need to drink less for weight management. Vitamin and mineral deficiencies occur commonly in heavy drinkers—in part because they lose their appetite for nutritious foods, but also because alcohol alters the absorption and use of some essential nutrients.

Key Points

- The Hassle Free Food Guide utilizes food groups to plan nutritionally sound food choices for health and weight loss.
- Foods are categorized into different food groups based on their food source and the nutrients they supply.
- All foods can be classified into five groups: Fruit and Vegetable Group; Grain Group; Milk Group; Meat Group; and the Other Category.
- Adults should have at least four servings from the Fruit-Vegetable Group, four servings from the Grain Group, two servings from the Milk Group, and two servings from the Meat Group daily. This suggested number of servings averages about 1,200 calories.
- Foods selected from the Other Category provide more calories than nutrients. These choices should be eaten in moderation.
- Favorite foods and family preferences should be considered when planning menus.
- The Dietary Guidelines provide a basis from which to make changes in eating habits for more healthful eating.

The Week Ahead

You have already been making a lot of changes in your eating behaviors and exercise habits. By all means, continue. Now is your chance to focus on your food choices. During the next week, modify your food choices closer to the number suggested in the Hassle Free Food Guide. Look over your food choices to see where recommendations from the Dietary Guidelines are possible.

Continue recording the same information in your *Log*. This week check the appropriate food group column for all the foods and beverages you consumed.

Action Plan

Goals

My goals for the week: _____

_____

_____

Goal-Setting

Plans for the week	Went well	Had problems	Keep practicing

Week in Review

The past week gave you a chance to begin getting your food choices in line. Take a few minutes to look over your *Log* and Action Plan. How did you do? Did you accomplish all your plans? Do some still need work? Think how your lifestyle and family preferences have been influencing your own food choices.

Rearranging and changing your food choices won't happen overnight. Like all the other weight management goals you are setting, they take continuous practice. Carry over plans related to managing your food choices to the next week's Action Plan.

Record your weight change on the Weight Graph. Total the time you spent exercising and calories used on the Exercise Log.

[1]U.S. Department of Agriculture & U.S. Department of Health, Education, and Welfare. (1980). *Nutrition and Your Health: Dietary Guidelines for Americans*. Washington, DC: U.S. Government Printing Office.

6: LOWERING YOUR CALORIES

Remember the old saying "look before you leap"? It's still good advice for anyone in a weight management program. Thinking and preplanning are cornerstones to weight management, especially when it comes to lowering calories. A little forethought can save you not only calories but the guilt and deprivation that usually accompany strict low calorie diets.

Weekly Calorie Deficit

The first step to lowering calories is to put "low" in perspective. Consider the calorie deficit you need in order to reach your weekly goal. If it takes 3,500 calories to lose a pound of fat, that would mean lowering your intake by 500 calories a day to lose 1 pound by the end of the week.

$$500 \text{ fewer kcal/day} \times 7 \text{ days} = 3,500 \text{ kcal deficit/week}$$

Depending upon what you're doing in the way of exercise, you might be able to lose a pound a week by lowering your intake by only 300 to 500 calories. Don't lose sight of your deficit figure. It helps make lowering calories more reasonable and attainable.

Strategies for Saving Calories

Lowering calories doesn't have to mean a future of bland and boring eating. The Four Ps listed here offer flexible and realistic strategies for saving calories. You can make changes in

1. **Portions**
2. **Preparation**
3. **Products**
4. **Passing**

The fourth strategy is based on the decision of whether you truly want and need the food. If your answer is *no*, you can always "pass." Once you feel confident in making eating behavior changes, passing may become one of your most personally satisfying decisions in weight management.

Portions

Most people underestimate how much they eat. Unless you've spent time measuring and weighing your food in the past, you may not be aware how your portions compare to recommended serving sizes.

It's common to base portion sizes on the size of a plate, a spoon, ladle, or scoop used to serve the food, and by habit—always dishing up the same amount. Small differences in portion sizes can make a big difference in saving calories.

Suggested serving size	Calories	Large serving size	Calories	Calorie savings
½ cup rice	70	Heaping ½ cup	115	**45**
Small scoop ice cream	130	Double dip	260	**130**
½ cup cottage cheese	110	Heaping ½ cup	135	**25**
1 Tbs peanut butter	94	Heaping Tbs	141	**47**
8 oz glass whole milk	150	Tall 12 oz glass	225	**75**
1 pat margarine	35	Chunk	98	**63**
10 peanuts	53	Handful	168	**115**
			Total calorie savings:	**500**

Tips for Managing Portions

- Base your serving sizes on average calorie values presented in each of the food groups in the Hassle Free Food Guide.
- Measure commonly eaten foods to get a better idea of your curent portion sizes.
- When eating at home, choose glasses and dishes that make your servings appear larger.
- Smaller cereal or salad bowls will make cereal portions appear larger.
- Use smaller dinner plates or salad plates to make smaller portions look larger. Plates with patterned or curved rims also make portions look larger.
- Using a smaller plate works well for salad bars and buffets. Although both salad bars and buffets offer choices for low-calorie eating, too much of a good thing can add up in calories.
- Use smaller serving utensils to dish out food.
- Serve food attractively. With very little effort, garnishes and pleasantly placed foods can make a plate look appealing. This is a portion-control technique that has worked well for many fine restaurants.
- Arrange food to give an illusion of more food. Spread food over a larger surface of the plate.
- Eat half the size portion you are now eating, especially for meat and meat dishes.
- Cutting portions in half holds true when eating out. Decide how much you are going to eat ahead of time, and ask for a doggie bag to take the rest home. Use your leftovers for another meal or planned snack.
- Leave some food on your plate as a signal to stop eating.

Preparation

The ingredients and preparation method affect the calorie content of a food. The extras added to foods—sour cream on baked potatoes, bacon bits on salad, and gravy or sauces on entrees—can be considered hidden calories. Once a food is prepared, trimming fat and removing poultry skins can also boost calorie savings.

| Food | Roasted | | | Batter Fried | | |
	With skin (or fat)	Without skin (trimmed)	Calorie savings	With skin	Without skin	Calorie savings
½ Chicken breast	193	142	**51**	360	161	**199**
1 Drumstick	112	76	**36**	193	82	**111**
3 oz Sirloin steak	329	176	**153**			

Tips for Managing Preparation

- Try new low-calorie recipes.
- If you reduce the amount of fat and sugar in your regular recipes, be prepared for changes in the product, especially in texture.
- Replace added butter and sauces on meats and vegetables with herbs and spices to enhance the natural flavor of foods.
- Switch to lower calorie cooking methods: broiling, baking, and barbecuing.
- Strip the fatty overcoat off meat and the skin off chicken before cooking.
- Avoid fried foods. Frying can take a low-calorie food and double or triple the calories.

1 medium baked potato = 104 kcal
20 french fries = 274 kcal

- Use a nonstick skillet for fat-free frying or sautéing.
- Roast and broil meats on a rack or grid to let fat drain from meat. This avoids cooking meat in its own fat.
- Refrigerate meat drippings, removing the hardened surface fat before using as gravy or au jus. Do the same for homemade soups.
- Tenderize leaner cuts of meat by marinating with fruit juices rather than oil and high sugar marinades.
- Sauté with vegetable and fruit juices.
- Avoid browning vegetables with meat. They tend to soak up a lot of fat.
- Steam vegetables.
- Cut back on hidden calories.

Food	Amount	Calories
Butter or margarine	1 tsp	35
Sugar	1 tsp	16
Sour cream	2 Tbs	62
Salad dressing	2 Tbs	75
Hollandaise sauce	2 Tbs	88
Cheese sauce	2 Tbs	38
Mayonnaise	2 Tbs	204
Whipped cream	2 Tbs	52

Products

Three ways to lower calories by making alternate food choices are as follows:

1. Select low-calorie alternatives for commonly eaten high-calorie favorites. Alternate fruit for frequently eaten heavy desserts.
2. Choose similar foods that give you a larger portion for the same number of calories. Different cereals vary greatly in calories for the same serving size.
3. Use reduced calorie or lowfat substitutes for commonly eaten foods. Lowfat dairy products offer an opportunity to save calories without sacrificing nutrition.

Tips for Managing Products

- If switching to lower calorie products brings you below a minimum calorie level for the Hassle Free Food Guide, increase the number of servings in the Fruit and Vegetable Group and the Grain Group to bring the figure back up to a safe level (1,200 kcal for women and 1,600 kcal for men). Eating less than 1,200 calories per day is nutritionally unsound.

Average fruit serving = 40 kcal

Average grain serving = 70 kcal

- Get the most food and nutrients for the least number of calories. Calories for the same measure can vary tremendously. Read the nutrition information panel to compare U.S. RDAs for equivalent calorie portions.

  Granola and bran type cereals as well as products with sugar coatings are usually higher in calories than puffed or plain flake cereals. Because bran type cereals are especially nutritious, it's important to adjust serving sizes appropriately to monitor calories.

Cereal	Amount	Calories
Puffed	1 cup	54
Flake	1 cup	110
Sugar-coated flakes	1 cup	160
Bran cereal	1 cup	144
Granola cereal	1 cup	520

- Investigate lower calorie substitutes for frequently eaten foods. Choosing lower calorie products lets you continue eating familiar foods, sometimes without having to reduce the portion size.

  The Hassle Free Food Guide milk group is based on whole milk. Substituting lower fat milk saves calories and lets you choose more servings from different groups.

Type of milk	Amount	Calories
Skim milk	1 cup	88
Buttermilk	1 cup	88
2% milk	1 cup	145
Whole milk	1 cup	150

- Choose lower fat products, including cheeses and lean ground beef, to lower the calories in mixed dishes, such as soups, casseroles, and Italian dishes.
- Choose lower percentages of fat in ground beef.

3 oz hamburger pattie (cooked) fat content	Calories
21%	235
10%	186
Calorie savings	**49**

- Well-marbled meats have more calories per pound than leaner cuts. Chuck roasts, round steak, and flank steak are leaner than sirloin, t-bone, and porterhouse steaks. Processed meats like sausage, cold cuts, and franks are relatively high in fat, sodium, and calories.
- It's not necessary to buy so-called diet foods. They are often more expensive than regular foods and in some cases don't save you that many calories.

2 Peach halves	Calories
"Diet"—in water	31
In natural fruit juice	45
In heavy syrup	78

- Reduce alcohol consumption and substitute lower calorie mixes in drinks. Club soda, mineral water, seltzer water, and diet sodas have very few or no calories.

Package Labeling

Package labeling is your window into foods. **Ingredient listings** give the ingredients according to weight, the more prominent ones coming first. Both ingredient listings and nutrition information found on most products may be used to compare similar products and alternate food choices.

Nutrition labeling is required for those products to which nutrients are added (such as cereals fortified with vitamins), products that make nutritional claims (such as "twice as much vitamin C as an orange"), or foods prepared for special dietary uses (such as those intended for infants or weight reduction). Many other products voluntarily carry nutrition labeling. The following sample label gives you an idea of what's on nutrition information labels.

Sample Label

Whole Wheat Bread
Nutrition Information

Serving Size . . . . 2 oz
(approx. 2 slices—actual slice thickness
and weight may vary slightly)

Servings Per Package 8

Calories 150
Protein . . . . 6 g
Carbohydrate . . . . 27 g
Fat . . . . 2 g

Percentage of U.S. Recommended Daily
Allowance (U.S. RDA)

Protein 10%
Vitamin A . . . . *
Vitamin C . . . . *
Thiamine (B$_1$) 15%
Riboflavin (B$_2$) 10%
Niacin 10%
Calcium 6%
Iron 10%

*Contains less than 2% of U.S. RDA of
these nutrients.

Nutrition information: Information must be given for a specified serving of the product as found in the container. This label shows information for a serving of whole wheat bread.

Calories: This lists the number of calories in one suggested serving and not the entire container unless the package contains only one manufacturer's suggested serving.

Serving (portion) sizes: This is the amount of food for which nutrition information is given. It may not be the same as the amount you eat.

Servings per container: This information can be very helpful in planning menus and controlling portion sizes.

Protein, carbohydrate, fat in weight by grams: The chapter on "Calculating Energy Costs" explained how to calculate the number of calories contributed by each of these nutrients. Remember, fat contributes more than twice as many calories per gram as protein and carbohydrate. The following calculations show how the final calorie figure was determined for two slices of whole-wheat bread. When calculating the calories contributed from each of these three nutrients, keep in mind that the figure you see printed on the label may actually be rounded off.

$$\begin{array}{r}
\text{Protein 4 kcal per g} \times 6 \text{ g} = 24 \text{ kcal} \\
\text{Carbohydrate 4 kcal per g} \times 27 \text{ g} = 108 \text{ kcal} \\
\underline{\text{Fat 9 kcal per g} \times 2 \text{ g} = 18 \text{ kcal}} \\
\text{Total calories per serving} = 150 \text{ kcal}
\end{array}$$

Percentage of U.S. Recommended Daily Allowance: The U.S. RDA for most nutrients is the highest Recommended Dietary Allowances of all sex/age categories. The male 17 to 19 age group has the highest requirement and is used as the standard for comparison.

Protein and seven vitamins and minerals must be shown in the same order as the sample label shows. Other vitamins and minerals may also be named. Space marked with an asterisk (*) indicates less than 2% of the nutrient. The food is a good source for a particular nutrient if it represents 15% or greater of the U.S. RDA. Listing amounts of fatty acids, cholesterol, and sodium is optional at this time.

When reading labels, watch for these terms:

- Lite or Light—There is no regulated definition for these terms. They don't necessarily mean the food is significantly lower in calories.
- Reduced Calorie—To carry this wording, the product must contain at least one-third fewer calories than traditional foods.
- Low Calorie—The product contains no more than 40 calories per serving.
- Lowfat—These foods contain less fat than their counterparts. This doesn't guarantee they are lower in calories, but most lowfat products are.
- Diet—This term has no consensus in definition.
- Sugar Free, Sugarless, No Sugar—These products do not contain sugar. This doesn't guarantee they are lower in calories.
- No Added Sugar—This phrase may be misleading. The food may already contain a high amount of natural carbohydrates, or it may be a food that traditionally doesn't have much sugar anyway. These products are not necessarily lower in calories.

Passing

Passing up food, especially if it's in the house and available, is just as difficult as passing it up in social situations. When at home, you can eat only what you or the shopper buys. Passing starts with some good "supermarket smarts" before and during grocery shopping.

Tips for Managing Passing

- Don't shop when you're hungry. Eat before you go. Tempting foods will be less tempting and you're less likely to nibble in the car on the way home if you shop on a full stomach.
- Start planning a week's worth of menus. Don't make a big deal about it. A little preplanning will save you hours in the long run. Once you have a general idea of what you're going to eat, you won't have to think constantly about food.
- Communicate your weight goals and Action Plans to the shopper and the person who prepares the meals. Be direct and tactful about changes you would like to make in your food choices. You'll be surprised how willing people are to help once you include them in your planning.
- Plan your favorite foods as well as other family preferences into the menu plans. Consider the Four Ps in your plans.
- If you have to buy snack foods for other members of the family, buy small individually packaged snacks. If you should open one yourself, at least you won't be eating a large bag.
- Try shopping without the kids or anyone else who might tempt you into buying things you really don't want.
- Make a shopping list and stick to it. From the moment you walk into the store, advertising and product labels are tempting you to buy.
- Use the Hassle Free Food Guide to plan your shopping list. Include a variety of foods from each food group.

Sample Hassle Free Shopping List

Item	Amounts
Fruits	
Vegetables	
Breads/cereals	
Dairy products	
Meat/poultry/fish/eggs/beans	
Other foods	
Condiments	
Household supplies	

Key Points

- Ways to save calories include controlling portion sizes, modifying preparation and cooking methods, and making lower calorie food choices.
- In some situations passing up a food that's not needed or wanted is the easiest way to save calories.
- When lowering calories brings you below the 1,200 calorie figure for women and 1,600 calorie level for men, additional servings from the Fruit and Vegetable Group and Grain Group should be added to maintain a nutritionally sound intake.

- Nutrition information and ingredient listings on product labels help you compare calories between similar products and make alternate food choices.
- Marketing techniques in the grocery store can make it hard to pass up tempting foods.

The Week Ahead

Continue exercising. Use your *Log* to identify high-calorie food choices in your eating. Select appropriate strategies for saving calories to practice during the next week. Refer to the Resource Shelf for recipe books on low-calorie cooking. Continue recording the times you eat, the degree of your hunger, the kind and amount of food you're eating, and the calories and food groups represented by your food choices. Write down your physical activity, and monitor your exercising heart rate immediately after exercise.

Action Plan

Goals

My goals for the week: _____

_____

_____

Goal-Setting

Plans for the week	Went well	Had problems	Keep practicing

Week in Review

At the end of the week, take a few minutes to look over your *Log* and Action Plan. How did you do? Did you accomplish all your plans? Do some still need work?

Based on your accomplishments, check the appropriate column on the Action Plan for all the plans you listed. If your plans went well, put a check in the first column. If you ran into problems, mark the second column and decide how you would do things differently. This may mean trying a different strategy or technique. Even if a technique worked well, you may want to continue working on it. Add any plans you need to carry over on your next week's Action Plan.

Record your weight change on the Weight Graph. Total the time you spent exercising and calories used on the Exercise Log.

Go through your past week's *Log* and list on the following chart the changes you made in food choices to lower calories.

Lowering Calories

1. List in the first column the foods you replaced.

2. Write in the second column substitutes or changes you made.

3. Estimate the number of calories you saved by making the change.

Foods/beverages	Changes made	Calories saved

7: MANAGING YOUR EATING BEHAVIORS

What makes you eat? You're the person who has to put food in your mouth, chew it, then swallow, but something usually happens shortly before you decide to eat. That something is called a *signal.* Eating, like most behavior, doesn't just happen. Signals are likely to trigger eating. How you respond to these signals affects weight management.

After keeping weight management *Logs* for several weeks, you are probably noticing some patterns in your eating behaviors. Any eye-openers?

As you repeat behaviors over and over and get some kind of encouragement or positive feedback, these behaviors usually become habit. For example, if each time you sit down to watch TV you settle in with a bag of chips and start to feel relaxed, you are likely to head for the TV again and continue nibbling away each time you want to unwind.

Behavior Chains

If you were to try to draw the sequence of events involved in an eating pattern, it would look much like a chain. One or more signals usually trigger a particular way of behaving, which is then followed by some kind of result. Behavior chains become a problem when they lead to overeating or inactivity.

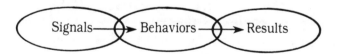

Signals——▶ Behaviors——▶ Results

Signals are cues or stimuli in the environment or our personal thoughts and feelings that trigger a particular way of behaving. Something as simple as the time of day, the smell of freshly baked bread, or a daydream about chocolate cake can be a signal to eat. The different categories in your *Log* represent potential signals for overeating: time of day, place where you eat, person or people you're with, how you feel, if you're hungry, and what you're eating.

Behaviors are what you do after receiving certain signals. A signal doesn't have to trigger you to eat right away. A lot of different behaviors can take place before eating actually occurs.

Results are what you get out of behaving a certain way. Some results make you feel good; others may bring on negative feelings like guilt. These "guilty" results can sometimes turn into signals themselves. Results that keep leading to eating are what sometimes start a vicious cycle of nonstop eating.

Your Signals

Use the information recorded in your *Log* to begin pinpointing possible signals leading to overeating. Look through each day's record. How often does each of these signals end up as problem eating? Check the column representing the frequency in which overeating is associated with the signal. For example, if when you feel bored, you notice that you consistently start nibbling, check the "Always" column.

Signals	Always	Sometimes (3 to 4 times/week)	Occasionally (1 to 2 times/week)
Time of day			
Where I am			
Who I'm with			
How I feel			
If I'm hungry			
Food itself			
Other signals			

Strategies for Modifying Eating Behaviors

During the past few weeks you started keeping *Logs* and have been setting goals and developing Action Plans to modify areas of eating and exercise that originally contributed to your weight problem.

The time to cope with a signal or problem situation is *before* you are faced with it. This takes planning. Knowing how to interrupt or alter a behavior chain and practicing these new behaviors contributes to successful weight management.

There are three major strategies for planning ways to interrupt or alter eating at key links in the behavior chain:

- **Delaying**
- **Substituting**
- **Avoiding**

Delaying

Adding time or steps between the links in the behavior chain gives you a chance to stop and rethink the situation. Delaying is especially effective if you think you are hungry but probably are not.

- Slow down the pace of eating.
- Do a relaxation exercise.

- Take the roundabout route to the kitchen or place where food is available.
- Preplan purchasing tempting foods. Buy them in a form that needs a lot of preparation (e.g., cake mix instead of a ready-made cake).
- Purchase individual snack packages so you have to open a new package each time you are considering a snack.
- Preplan what foods you are going to eat, and fill in your *Log* before you eat.
- Store tempting foods so they are difficult to get at. Locations like high shelves, the freezer, bottom shelves in the refrigerator are good spots.
- Put off unplanned eating as long as possible. Make yourself do something else like mail a letter or brush your teeth before you eat.

Substituting

Substituting is a way to actually break a behavior chain. It replaces eating with another activity, something enjoyable. Doing something enjoyable is likely to give a positive reinforcement to a "new" activity. These new activities must be incompatible with eating, ones that won't eventually lead to eating. Switching back to eating should be difficult—almost impossible—while doing the new activity.

When selecting new activities, keep in mind they must be readily available and be able to compete with the urge to eat. There are two groups of activities that meet these criteria:

- **Pleasant activities**—Doing hobbies, walking around the block, working in the garden, reading a good book, listening to music, taking a leisurely bath, sleeping
- **Necessary activities**—Running errands, cleaning the house, making phone calls, going through your office in-box, opening mail, doing household projects, paying bills

Make your own list of activities you like to do and those you must do. Refer to the list whenever you feel the urge to eat. Another technique is to write each activity on a slip of paper and drop it in a cookie jar. Instead of reaching for food, open the jar and pull out an activity.

Substitute Activities

Things I like to do:

_____

_____

_____

_____

_____

_____

_____

Things I have to do:

_____

_____

_____

_____

_____

_____

_____

_____

Avoiding

There are some situations when delaying or substituting is so difficult that avoiding the situation altogether may be the best answer. Making food less visible or accessible is another way to lessen the likelihood that a behavior chain will occur.

- Minimize your contact with food. Try not to go near the kitchen or lounge area at work.
- Avoid bringing tempting foods into the house in the first place.
- If problems occur while eating with a particular person, try to avoid eating with that person. Plan nonfood activities together.
- Spend your free time or coffee breaks away from food.
- Make food available only for meals and planned snacks.
- Make eating a single activity. Avoid eating while doing other things like reading the paper, watching TV, or driving.
- If you don't have to be in the kitchen when food is being prepared, get out.
- Ask other family members to prepare their own snacks and lunches.
- Store foods only in storage locations. Avoid keeping food in desk drawers, glove compartments, nightstands, and other nonstorage locations around the house.
- Serve meals from the kitchen or buffet. Avoid putting serving bowls on the table.
- If foods are placed on the table during meals, set them out of reach or on the opposite end of the table.
- Remove dishes as soon as possible after eating.
- Scrape food directly into the garbage or disposal after clearing.
- Wrap leftovers immediately after a meal, and store in the refrigerator or freezer.
- Incorporate leftovers in planned snacks or meals.

Food Storage and Eating Locations: Floor Plan

Identifying where food is stored and how the availability of food triggers your eating will make you more aware of these signals. After completing this Floor Plan activity, decide how you could change either the availability of food or the locations where you eat in order to manage your eating behaviors better.

1. Using the floor plan space below, draw a plan of your house. Be sure to draw in all rooms, including bedrooms, the playroom, basement, patio, garage, and so on.
2. Place an "x" in each location where food is usually available or stored, both at home and outside your house. If you're not sure, take a quick tour of your house. **Don't forget your car, office, and other places outside your house.**
3. Refer to your past week's *Log*. Go through each day's record, noting the locations where you ate meals or snacks or found yourself nibbling. Include eating out at restaurants or a friend's house.
4. For every time you ate, place an M (meal), S (snack), or N (nibbling) in the locations on your floor plan where eating occurred.

Rewarding New Behaviors

Think of why you turn to food in different situations. Eating was a positive reinforcer, your reward. Part of weight management is developing new behaviors, then rewarding them appropriately so they are likely to be repeated the next time a similar situation arises. Rewarding yourself for new behaviors is a tremendous motivator.

It's a good idea to encourage support from other people, but it's even more important to start rewarding yourself. Unfortunately, giving ourselves rewards isn't easy, mainly because we feel awkward and uncomfortable about doing something nice for ourselves.

New behaviors must be reinforced in order to become habits. Knowing you can't always count on other people to give you the reinforcement you need may be an incentive to look to yourself for rewards. You are the most reliable and dependable source of rewards.

There are many types of rewards. The key is to decide what you want and what will strongly reinforce a new behavior.

Money

There are different ways to use money for a reward. A lump sum can be set aside to be used once you reach certain goals. Money can be set aside each time you achieve a short-term goal or implement a specific technique. It accumulates for a special purchase, something you could never justify spending money on, or for a special occasion: a day trip, a vacation, or an evening at the theater.

Activities

Reward yourself by doing something you rarely have time for or take time to do because of family, home, or job responsibilities. Your family will need to help with some of these rewards. Here are some suggestions:

- Take a half day or day and go shopping for yourself.
- Take time and go to a good movie or to visit friends.
- Ask a family member to take over one of your responsibilities for 2 days: cutting the lawn, raking leaves, doing housework.
- Spend time on a favorite hobby.
- Set aside time to read a book you've been wanting to read.
- Call a special friend long distance!
- Subscribe to a new magazine.

Thoughts

How we think and feel about ourselves may be the most beneficial rewards. General thoughts about ourselves influence our self-images. Specific thoughts linked to particular behaviors need to be developed, remembered, and repeated.

After substituting an old behavior with a new nonfood activity, thoughts like "It feels great to finish this project" or "I feel terrific now that I've walked" reinforce the replacement activity.

My Reward List

Refer to your goals and Reward List every day. If you accomplish areas on your Action Plan for the day, reward yourself. In order to get into the habit of rewarding yourself, check whether you rewarded yourself or not on the *Log*.

1. Decide which accomplishments you want to reward and list them as specific goals and plans in the first column. These accomplishments should include your goals and plans for making changes in physical activity, eating behaviors, food choices, and weight changes. Feel free to be as specific or as general as you like.
2. In the space to the right of what you want to reward, list specific ways to reward yourself. For example, if your plan is to avoid eating in the car on the way home from work, your reward for not eating in the car for a specified number of days might be going to see a favorite movie on the weekend.

Goals and plans	Rewards

Key Points

- Signals in the environment, your own thoughts and feelings, and how other people respond to you can trigger eating.
- An eating behavior pattern is like a chain. Signals trigger a certain way of behaving, which is then followed by a result that may or may not encourage the behavior to occur again.
- To avoid overeating, you may interrupt or alter behavior chains.
- Adding time between signals may delay eating. Substituting other activities for eating and avoiding or lessening exposure to food will interfere with a behavior chain.
- Rewards are needed to reinforce new behaviors and increase the likelihood they will occur again in the future.

The Week Ahead

Keep up the good work! Continue exercising. Start using exercise as a substitute activity for unplanned eating. Based on your specific signals, select strategies from the three lists to try out and practice during the next week. Make sure to reward yourself for changes in both eating and exercise behaviors.

In addition to recording physical activity and your exercising heart rate, complete the first six columns of your *Log*. As you accomplish your goals and plans, make sure to check whether you rewarded yourself.

Action Plan

Goals

My goals for the week: _____

_____

_____

Goal-Setting

Plans for the week	Went well	Had problems	Keep practicing

Week in Review

At the end of the week, take a few minutes to look over your *Log* and Action Plan. How did you do? Did you accomplish all your plans? Do some still need work?

Based on your accomplishments, check the appropriate column on the Action Plan for all the plans you listed. If your plans went well, put a check in the first column. If you ran into problems, mark the second column and decide how you would do things differently. This may mean trying a different strategy or technique. Even if a technique worked well, you may want to continue working on it. Add any plans you need to carry over on your next week's Action Plan.

Record your weight on the Weight Graph and total the time you spent exercising and calories used on the Exercise Log.

In addition to evaluating your Action Plan to see how strategies worked during the week, follow these instructions as you complete the following chart.

Strategy Check

- List all the strategies you tried in order to interrupt or alter your behavior chains.
- Write a brief description of the situation when the strategies were used. For example, you decided to take a short walk during your break to avoid nibbling on doughnuts left in the lounge. In this example, you "substituted" another activity for potential eating and also "avoided" the location by going someplace else.
- In the "How did they work?" column, indicate how each strategy worked by placing a "+" if it worked or "−" if it didn't.

Strategies I used	When	How did they work?

8: BUILDING SUCCESS TEAMS

HELP WANTED: Tactful supporters desired to assist in weight management efforts. Must be willing to reinforce, listen, motivate, and know when to leave well enough alone. Knowledge of lyrics from "With a Little Help From My Friends" and "Bridge Over Troubled Water" a plus.

With all the people you know, you'd think it would be easy to build a team of supporters to reinforce your weight loss efforts. It's not. A lot of time and effort is required, but the results are well worth it.

People often hinder weight management, many times unknowingly. The smiling face behind the fast-food counter trying to add some french fries or an apple turnover to your order, or a loving spouse presenting a box of chocolates in celebration of reaching your weight goal—both are innocent, but a challenge to your efforts all the same.

Through the *Logs* you've probably picked up several signals and behavior patterns involving other people. There may be situations when other people had something to do with your food choices, eating behaviors, or exercise plans. Take a few minutes to stop and look through your *Log* right now. Start to get a feel for who some of these people are and how they are doing it.

Building a Team

One way to be successful in achieving your weight management goals is to draw on a network of supportive relationships for help. You may already have "success teams" for support in other aspects of your life. Some of these same people will become part of your weight management success team. The requests you ask of them may be different, some even difficult for them to adjust to at first. Part of the building process involves changing the way others relate to you and how you in turn relate to them.

It's important to appreciate that once you develop a success team, you are still the one in control of your own decisions and actions. Use the team for support, not as a crutch or an excuse.

Four Steps to Success

Some people set themselves up for failure by being unreasonable in their requests or by not communicating their needs to success team members. Knowing how to go about building a team and then taking the steps to *do it* will move you closer to achieving your weight management goals.

Step 1: Identify Your Success Team Members

A well-developed support team includes a variety of individuals. It's not limited to people who are just close to you or who are good at listening or at giving advice. It includes people who directly affect your weight management efforts as well as those from whom you can learn in achieving your goals. Family, friends, co-workers, outsiders, and spiritual supporters are potential members. Don't forget yourself as a key member.

The following list illustrates potential success team members:

- **Role models**—Someone who successfully manages his or her weight may be a role model. Role models not only show what is possible but are resources of valuable tips and information.
- **Common interests**—People who share common interests or concerns can be especially important in keeping you motivated and in helping to tackle problems. Someone who enjoys physical activity and is willing to exercise with you would be a plus to your team. Seek out people with whom you can do nonfood activities. Members from your weight management group are ideal candidates for membership on your team.
- **Close friends**—People who help provide emotional support, who may enjoy some of the same interests, and who can keep you from becoming isolated and alienated are a great help. Family members are part of this group.
- **Helpers**—People who can be depended upon in a crisis to provide assistance should be included.
- **Challengers**—People who keep you on your toes are important. Due to the way they respond to you, they motivate you to develop new skills and new ways of doing things. Challengers may also be people who hinder your efforts, either intentionally or unintentionally. They may want to see you lose weight, but not at the expense of taking away from their own needs. Your aim should be to change how they respond to you.

Step 2: Identify the Kind of Support You Need

Each member is likely to offer different kinds of support. Besides seeking emotional support and encouragement, you might want to solicit help in practicing some of the techniques learned in the program or in achieving your exercise goals.

The request made of a member must be specific (e.g., clear dishes, prepare own snacks, give compliments, don't offer food).

Step 3: Evaluate Your Expectations of Others

Your requests for support should be in the form of behaviors the other person is willing to do and capable of performing. Expectations should be reasonable and equitable. It's important that the relationship be one in which both sides feel there is a fair arrangement, whether it be accomplished by returning help or whatever else makes sense. Guilt can easily build up when there is a feeling of indebtedness that cannot be repaid. You also want positive support, not resentment from the other person.

To help evaluate your expectations, ask these questions about each person and the requests you're making:

"Am I overloading one or two people with demands?"

"Can the person handle the responsibility of becoming involved in my efforts?" For personal reasons, some people may feel they can't take on more responsibilities at this time. Others may not want to get involved for fear of letting you down.

"Am I asking for something they can give?" These may be changes in their current behavior or food choices, emotional support, time, or money. Even though your supporters may be ready and willing, they may not be capable of providing what you ask.

"Will the person benefit from helping me?"

Step 4: Communicate Your Feelings and Needs

Your expectations must be communicated to the people from whom you are asking support. This is where support systems fail. It's often difficult to ask someone for help. At first feelings of guilt, timidness, or pride stand in the way. Remember, people cannot read your mind. They have to be told what you want them to do, even if it's as basic as letting people know you are trying to lose weight.

Many of the behaviors you are changing—eating slower or limiting your meals to one location—are not obvious. People around you will not know to compliment you for eating less or pausing during the meal unless they know your goals. Here are some tips to keep in mind when communicating:

* **Be assertive**—Practice being direct in stating what you want and saying no.
* **Be open**—Be tactful, but say what's on your mind.
* **Be specific**—Help others understand what they should do. State how you would like to see behaviors change.
* **Be consistent**—Don't give a mixed message by turning down something to eat one day and accepting it the next. If you say you're going to exercise, don't give excuses every time you're not in the mood.
* **Be positive**—Approach your communication with enthusiasm and willingness to commit yourself to weight management.
* **Be thankful**—Compliment your support person for paying attention to you and helping you out.

My Success Team

Use the following chart to start identifying success team members and how you would like them to support your weight management goals.

1. List potential team members.
2. Identify the kind of support you want from each member. Be specific.
3. Evaluate your requests by asking yourself if they are reasonable. If they are, put a "+" in the third column. If they are not, make adjustments in your requests so they become more reasonable.
4. Decide if you communicated your desires to the other person. If yes, put a "+" in the last column. If no, leave the space blank until you orally communiate these desires.

Team members	What am I asking?	Is it reasonable?	Did we communicate?

Your Best Supporter: You

Chapter 7 brought out the importance of reinforcing your new behaviors. Part of this positive reinforcement comes from including yourself on your success team. The way you communicate your expectations to yourself, or your "self-talk," has a lot to do with self-esteem and long-term success.

Self-talk is what you tell yourself: your thoughts and feelings about the kind of person you are and what you can or can't do. Positive self-talk conversations focus on realistic and logical thoughts about weight management and your capabilities. They're the pat on the back and pep talks we all need. Negative thoughts are loaded with excuses and show a defeatist attitude. They can be more destructive and challenging than a real life situation.

You know weight management takes a lot of effort. It's not unusual to try to talk yourself out of practicing techniques or keeping records. Most self-talk falls into five different categories depending on how it relates to your overall weight management efforts: weight loss, capabilities, excuses, standards, and food thoughts. Start countering your own negative self-talk with more positive thoughts. Practice saying the new thoughts to yourself.

Self-Talk

Negative thoughts	Positive thoughts
Weight loss	
"This weight isn't coming off fast enough."	"This isn't a race. It took years to put on the weight. I'm going to take each day at a time. Changes in my eating and exercise habits are going to pay off in the long run."
"I'm eating the same as Alice, and she's losing faster. It's just not fair."	"Each person is different. I'm not going to worry about other people. I'm proud of myself."
Capabilities	
"I just don't have the will-power."	"There's no such thing as 'will-power,' just poor planning. I'm going to learn from my mistakes. I know how to pick up the pieces."
"I'll probably just regain it again."	"I feel terrific. I like the new me. I'm never looking back."
Excuses	
"I can't lose weight; I have to eat what my wife cooks."	"I'm going to ask my wife to help. She's a great cook, and together we should be able to think of ways to change our eating so everyone is happy."
"I can't lose weight with a schedule like mine."	"My schedule isn't any worse than anyone else's. I need to be a little more creative in how I plan my eating and exercise. Weight management means a lot to me."
Standards	
"I cheated; that does it for the day."	"Why should one sweet or extra portion blow it for me? I just need to cut back somewhere else."
"I went off my diet. I feel so guilty."	"Feeling guilty never changes anything. I've made a lot of progress. I'm proud of myself."
"I paid for it; I'd better eat it."	"I'm eating out because I enjoy the company or it's convenient. That's what I'm paying for."
Food thought	
"All I think about is food."	"I'm an intelligent person. I can switch the topic to something else."
"When I go grocery shopping, tempting foods seem to jump off the shelf at me. I can't think rationally about what I'm doing."	"I know supermarkets stock tempting foods in certain locations. I'll make sure I'm not hungry when I go shopping, and stick to my list."

Key Points

* People can influence weight management goals in a positive or negative way.
* Building a team of supportive relationships doesn't happen overnight. A lot of time and effort is required.
* When building a success team, identify realistic ways people can help and tell them what you would like them to do.
* Give your team members positive reinforcement for their support.
* Self-talk is a way to reinforce yourself as a team member.

The Week Ahead

Continue practicing techniques in your Action Plan to reinforce your weight management goals. Start reevaluating how you would relate to other people and what requests or expectations you have of them. Work on communicating your goals more effectively to potential success team members. Become more conscious of the thoughts and feelings you have about yourself. Begin converting some of your negative self-talk to more positive thoughts.

During the next week, record when and where you're eating, who is with you and how you feel at the time, and what and how much you're eating. Continue to list your exercise and heart rate, and check to see if you're rewarding yourself for accomplishments.

Action Plan

Goals

My goals for the week: _____

_____

_____

Goal-Setting

Plans for the week	Went well	Had problems	Keep practicing

Week in Review

Many of your accomplishments this past week involved other people. How did things go? Use last week as a starting point from which to continue your open and honest communication with other people.

Take a few minutes to look over your *Log* and Action Plan. Evaluate how things went, and carry over plans into next week's Action Plan. Record your weight change on the Weight Graph and total the time you spent exercising and calories used on the Exercise Log.

9: MANAGING SPECIAL SITUATIONS

Eating out is no excuse to "blow it big," especially when eating away from home is becoming the rule rather than the exception. More than one out of three meals is eaten outside the home. Add to this eating during parties or while traveling, and it becomes more obvious why eating out is a real challenge to weight management.

To manage special situations, treat eating as you would at home. **Plan ahead** and **be reasonable**. Signals while eating away from home are a little different, but you can still control what you put into your mouth, even if you aren't the cook.

Four common and challenging situations facing weight management are eating at fancy restaurants or fast-food places, office eating, eating at parties, and eating while traveling. This chapter deals with suggestions for ways to manage these special eating situations. Each situation affects different people differently. As you read through this chapter, decide which tips might help you out with your particular problems. Add these suggestions to your Action Plan for the upcoming week.

Managing Eating Out

More guilt than enjoyment can accompany eating out for the weight-conscious eater. This doesn't have to be the case. If eating out is part of your lifestyle, *plan ahead* for it and *be reasonable*. The following suggestions may be helpful.

Plan ahead:

- Don't wait until the last minute to decide to eat out. Make your decision early so you can plan food choices for the entire day.
- Space your eating throughout the day. Don't skip meals. Eat a little lighter, saving servings from food groups for the meal out.
- Screen restaurants ahead of time. Find out which ones offer a variety of foods and low-calorie preparation methods.
- Avoid busy times when you know you'll have to wait to be seated or served. Long waits when you're hungry may lead to overeating signals.
- Plan what you're going to order and eat before entering the restaurant. Spend as little time as possible looking over the menu.
- Use your *Log* to preplan food choices. Jot down what you will order ahead of time. When you're finished, check to see how close you came to eating only your original choices.
- Once you make your menu decision, stick to it. Don't let waiters coax you to change your mind.
- If out for a business lunch or dinner, let others order first. Your choice won't seem as obvious, and customers and colleagues won't feel obligated to change their minds because of your decision.
- Try to exercise before going out. This helps take the edge off your appetite and will help use some of the extra calories you are about to eat.
- If you are going to eat later than usual, plan a light snack so you won't be starved and tempted to nibble as soon as you are seated.

- Fast food doesn't mean you have to eat it quickly. If you eat slowly, you are less likely to go back for a second "meal."
- Make sure take-out food makes it home. Put it in the trunk so you won't be tempted to nibble.

Be reasonable:

- Practice the Four Ps.
- Portions are usually large. Divide entrees in half, especially meat.
- Be leery of "diet plates." Most are higher in calories, especially fat calories, than other items on the menu.
- When finished, move your plate to the side and tell the waiter you would like a doggie bag for leftovers.
- Restaurants are accustomed to special requests. Order meat, fish, and poultry baked or broiled. Ask for it plain—without butter, gravy, or sauces.
- Watch for hidden calories.
- Move crackers, corn chips, and rolls out of reach. If your eating companion agrees, ask the waiter to remove them.
- Trim visible fats from meat.
- Be reasonable with extras you add to low-calorie vegetables, including salads and potatoes.
- Choose lower calorie favorites. If entrees are high-calorie, consider ordering two appetizers. Ask the waiter to serve them as the main course.
- Don't end up sipping all your calories. Alcohol, soft drinks, and several cups of coffee with cream and sugar boost the day's caloric intake.
- If you pass on a favorite, be prepared to live with that decision. If you feel you're being deprived, you might end up eating twice the calories after returning home.
- If you have your heart set on dessert, be reasonable. Decide to split one with a friend or make a point of asking for only a half portion.
- Appendix E offers guidelines and caloric values for different restaurant menus. Refer to them to learn more about different eating out food choices.

Managing Office Eating

If you spend a large percentage of your day at the office, it's reasonable to expect some special eating challenges. Food may be easily available, perhaps too available. A box of doughnuts open in the lounge or someone's baking creation sitting out for the office to taste may be prime targets for a hungry person having a bad day. Use the following suggestions to help you plan ahead and be reasonable at the office.

Plan ahead:

- Use your *Log* and desk calendar to space eating throughout the day.
- Start with something to eat in the morning. If breakfast is a problem, take a snack to eat when you arrive at work or during an early break.
- Keep a list of "reasonable" restaurants to frequent with customers and colleagues. Be the first to suggest a place so you can stay in control of the food choices.

Be reasonable:

- Identify work situations that may be leading to overeating. Practice strategies for managing behavior chains at the office.
- Schedule breaks throughout the day, even if they are just to get up and stretch.
- Get away from your desk at lunch. Use part of your lunch time to walk, relax, and refresh your thinking for the rest of the day.

- Doughnuts, baked goods, and candy are high in calories and low in nutrients. Don't consider having these extras unless you can afford the calories. Bring in low-calorie snacks to eat during breaks.
- Have more fun, not more calories, at office parties. Be moderate in alcohol consumption.
- Plan to do all eating away from your desk. Food stashed in drawers often signals eating. If you eat while doing work or another activity, you are more likely to eat quickly and still feel hungry.
- If you find yourself nibbling on snacks left out in the coffee lounge, stay away from the area.
- Steer clear of vending machines and snack carts if the foods are too tempting.

Managing Party-Time Eating

Social eating, whether you are out at a party or entertaining at home, usually goes one of two ways. Most people are on their best behavior while around others, or they use this as an excuse for a last fling before "starting a diet tomorrow." One of the major problem areas to control during social situations is available food. Food is usually everywhere and within easy reach. So at parties, it's especially important to plan ahead in order to be reasonable.

Plan ahead:

- Space your eating throughout the day.
- Don't go out hungry. If the party is late, have a light snack before leaving home.
- Offer to bring something. Fresh vegetable trays and low-calorie dips will be appreciated by all. Most people have diet sodas on hand, but just in case take a few bottles.
- If you are entertaining, you can control both the food and the activities. Plan nonfood activities so food doesn't become the center of focus. Control the amount of available food left out for nibbling.
- After arriving at a party, try to get a feel for when food will be officially served. You don't want to eat all your calories early in the evening only to discover the full spread won't be out until midnight.

Be reasonable:

- For buffets and cocktail parties, survey the available food before eating. Make very conscious decisions on what you want to and will eat.
- When taking food, place small portions on a plate or napkin, then move as far away from the food as possible.
- Try not to stand or sit near snacks. If you find yourself staring at a bowl of nuts, inconspicuously move them out of reach.
- Make conscious decisions on the type and amount of snacks you will eat.
- Be careful not to get into a vicious circle of eating salty snacks, getting thirsty, and sipping away your calories on alcohol and soft drinks.
- Set a limit on alcoholic drinks before you get to the party. After your limit, switch to club soda, mineral water, or diet soda with a twist of lemon or lime.

Managing Travel Eating

Any kind of travel—vacation or business—adds greater challenges because it usually combines several of the other special situations as well. There is no reason why weight management cannot continue while you're traveling. More and more hotels are catering to health-conscious guests with lighter fare menus and exercise facilities. Here are some ways you can plan ahead to be reasonable when traveling.

Plan ahead:

- Continue keeping your *Logs* and practicing techniques written in your Action Plans.
- Consider ordering lower calorie menu choices for plane travel. Special meals can be ordered 24 hours prior to travel from most major airlines.

- Incorporate strategies for managing your eating time and spacing eating throughout the day. Eating times may be more difficult to manage on vacation, especially if meals are served only at set times.
- During long car trips, plan scheduled breaks for both eating and exercising.
- If you anticipate having difficulty finding restaurants with low-calorie selections, pack some meals and snacks.
- Try to avoid nibbling constantly while in the car. Store food in a cooler in the trunk.

Be reasonable.

- Most restaurant meals, due to preparation methods, will have more calories than you normally eat. This is another reason why it's important to make everything you put into your mouth count.
- Pass up ''unconscious'' calories: peanuts before dinner on the plane and mints after dinner on the way out of the restaurant.
- Plan your traveling hours so you aren't caught short of sleep. Feeling tired, anxious, or rushed could become signals leading to problem eating.
- Incorporate in your travel reasonable tips suggested for eating out and eating socially.

Key Points

- Principles of weight management similar to those used at home can be applied to special eating situations.
- Steps to plan ahead and make reasonable food choices help control eating away from home.
- Knowing more about the caloric and nutritional value of different foods helps in making reasonable decisions.

The Week Ahead

Continue your exercise plans. Based on your schedule for the week ahead, select several techniques to manage upcoming special situations. Remember to set aside time to review your *Log* each night and to practice different relaxation techniques demonstrated in class.

During the next week, record when and where you are eating, how hungry you are and who you're with, and what you are eating and how much. Start checking which food groups your food choices represent.

Action Plan

Goals

My goals for the week: _____

_____

_____

Goal-Setting

Plans for the week	Went well	Had problems	Keep practicing

Week in Review

At the end of the week, take a few minutes to look over your *Log* and Action Plan. Did you experience any special situations? Were any of the strategies suggested helpful?

Based on how things went, check the appropriate column on the Action Plan for all the plans you listed. Carry over plans to work on changes in your food choices, eating behaviors, and exercise habits. Look back over your past Action Plans for ideas.

Record your weight change on the Weight Graph and total the time you spent exercising and calories used on the Exercise Log.

10: CONTINUING YOUR COMMITMENT

Take a deep breath. Put a smile on your face. *You've made it!*

The past weeks have brought with them much self-evaluation and change. You are about to enter a new phase: living a lifetime with successful weight management. If you still have goals to reach, tackle them with determination and enthusiasm. If you're setting out to maintain your losses, do so with conviction for your new lifestyle.

My Achievements

Take a few minutes to look back at where you were when you started the program and to look at where you are now. Flip through the chapters; check over past Action Plans, your Eating and Lifestyle Questionnaire, and your Weight Profile. Jot down before and after comments showing changes.

Where was I when I started?

Weight:

Exercise habits:

Caloric intake:

Food choices:

Eating behaviors:

Where am I now?

Weight:

Exercise habits:

Caloric intake:

Food choices:

Eating behaviors:

My Success Team:

Feelings about myself:

How do you feel about your achievements? Your progress in the program is not measured by losses in weight and body fat alone. Changing exercise habits, eating behaviors, and food choices, as well as relationships with other people, are also accomplishments. The bottom line is how you feel about yourself and the responsibilities and commitments you've made to become a healthier and happier person.

A Lifetime of Success

The *Y's Way to Weight Management* is a program you don't stop. Your willingness to change shows a lifetime commitment to weight management. You now have a solid foundation on which to keep adding achievements. Weekly action planning helped map out strategies for achieving long- and short-term goals. Continue reevaluating your eating and lifestyle goals and planning strategies for dealing with different situations as they occur.

Writing down where you would like your weight management goals to take you and planning how you get there helps continue your successes. Give some serious thought to shaping your future as you complete the Long-Term Action Plan.

Long-Term Action Plan

Date: _____

Goals for:

* Weight

    In one month I want to be _____

    In two months I want to be _____

    In three months I want to be _____

    In four months I want to be _____

    In five months I want to be _____

    In six months I want to be _____

    In *one year* I want to be _____

* Eating behaviors

    _____

    _____

* Exercise

    _____

    _____

* Food choices

    _____

    _____

Goal-setting steps I will take:

1. _____

2. _____

3. _____

4. _____

5. _____

6. _____

Obstacles I can expect: _____

_____

_____

Rewards for achieving my goals: _____

_____

Three Cheers for Motivation

There are many ways to keep the momentum of your weight management efforts moving. Ongoing support groups, involvement in exercise and fitness classes, and new projects and classes to expand your interests and talents are steps in the right direction. Staying on top of your priorities and goals will keep your motivation high as you move through new phases of weight management. Like anything else, staying motivated doesn't come easily. Here are three steps to help keep you motivated.

Step 1: Keep Weight Management a High Priority

Weight management jumped to a high-priority ranking when you started the program. Keep it there. It is understandable that unexpected life events will come up and you may have to shift priorities for a while. Look at shifts as temporary. Remind yourself you have learned the skills to manage eating. You won't forget them.

Decide to manage your eating behaviors as well as possible, even if food choices slip during setbacks. Above all, keep exercising. When problems are resolved, start concentrating on your weight management efforts again, boosting weight management back to the top of your list.

Step 2: Keep Checking Your Goals

As you accomplish goals, start planning steps to achieve new ones. Be realistic. No one is totally in control or totally out of control of anything. If you are having difficulty with a goal, break it down into smaller, more manageable goals. Keep in mind that certain times are better than others for tackling a particular goal. Be flexible.

Once you reach your weight goal, gradually increase your caloric intake. Increase the number of servings to reflect a 100-calorie per day increase. If after a week, you are still losing, add another 100 calories. If you gain, cut back. Eventually your weight will stabilize.

Step 3: Keep Tabs on Your Accomplishments

Up to now your weekly *Logs* and Action Plans helped you keep a close eye on your progress. Continue keeping *Logs*. Once you reach most of your goals, cut back recording to every other week, then one week a month. Pick one or two areas to monitor. If you find yourself slipping, start recording again on a regular basis.

Come up with some early warning signs that will let you know if things are slipping. The obvious one is weighing yourself. When you get a warning, do something immediately. Don't put it off!

Congratulations!

Keep smiling. You should be proud of yourself. Don't forget to share your accomplishments with your Success Team.

This book has been written and designed so you can continue using it even after you finish the final chapter. Keep referring to the Hassle Free Food Guide and special charts throughout the book and appendices and you'll find continuing your commitment to weight management is a rewarding, positive part of your lifestyle.

A: EATING AND LIFESTYLE QUESTIONNAIRE

Answer the questions based on what you are doing now.

1. How many meals a day do you eat? _____

2. Which meals do you regularly skip? _____

3. What time do you usually eat your meals?

   Breakfast _____ Lunch _____ Dinner _____

4. At what times do you snack during the day or night? _____

   _____

5. Would you consider yourself a fast or slow eater?

   _____ fast   _____ slow

6. Where do you usually eat? List all the locations.

   _____   _____

   _____   _____

   _____   _____

   _____   _____

7. Whom do you eat with? List names of people.

   _____   _____

   _____   _____

   _____   _____

   _____   _____

   Go back over your list and put a "+" next to those people who either strongly encourage you to eat or seem to bring out your urge to eat.

8. What moods seem to bring out your urge to eat?

   _____

   _____

9. Who does the food shopping? _____

10. Is a shopping list used? _____ yes   _____ no   _____not sure

11. List all the foods you feel are tempting.

    _____   _____

    _____   _____

    _____   _____

    _____   _____

    _____   _____

    _____   _____

    Put a "+" next to the foods you think are contributing to your weight problem.

    Circle all the foods in your home now. Also put a circle around foods stored in your desk at work or in your car.

12. Do you think you eat a balanced diet? _____ yes   _____ no

13. Where would you rate the amount of physical activity you perform while at work? Put an "X" along the line.

    very little   little   moderate   active   very active
    _____

14. Where would you rate the amount of physical activity you perform during your leisure time? Put an "X" along the line.

    very little   little   moderate   active   very active
    _____

15. How physically fit do you feel? Put an "X" along the line.

    unfit   below average   average   above average   very fit
    _____

B: ACTIVITY AND FITNESS BENEFITS CHART

For the purposes of this chart, activities are rated from very good (the highest ranking), to poor (the lowest).

| Activity | Aerobic benefits | Muscle strength and endurance | | Flexibility |
		Upper body	Lower body	
Aerobic dance	Very good	Fair	Very good	Very good
Basketball	Good	Fair	Good	Fair
Canoeing	Good to fair	Good	Poor	Poor
Cross-country skiing	Very good	Good	Good	Good
Cycling	Very good	Poor	Very good	Poor
Downhill skiing	Fair	Good	Good	Good
Golf	Fair	Fair	Fair	Fair
Handball	Good	Good	Good	Fair
Racquetball	Good	Good	Good	Fair
Running	Very good	Fair	Very good	Poor
Squash	Good	Good	Good	Fair
Swimming	Very good	Very good	Good	Good
Tennis	Good	Good	Good	Good
Volleyball	Good to fair	Fair	Good to fair	Fair
Walking (briskly)	Good	Poor	Fair	Poor

C: NUTRIENT CHART

Vitamins

Vitamin A (Soluble in Fat)

Primary Sources—Dark green leafy vegetables, yellow fruits and vegetables; liver; butter and fortified margarine; cream, whole milk, and cheeses made from whole milk

Main Roles—Aids bone and teeth formation; helps form normal outer and inner skin (mucous membranes); enhances night and color vision

If Deficient—Poor bone and teeth development; deterioration of outer and inner skin; night blindness, blindness, drying of the eyes

If Overdosed—Drying and peeling of skin, rashes; loss of hair; bone and joint pain, fragile bones; enlarged liver and spleen; brain and nervous system injury; insomnia; menstrual irregularities; yellowing of skin (from carotene-containing foods—carrots)

Vitamin D (Soluble in Fat)

Primary Sources—Fortified milk; egg yolk; fish liver oils; sardines, salmon, tuna; direct exposure of skin to sunlight

Main Roles—Regulates intestinal absorption of calcium and phosphorous; takes a part in protein metabolism; aids in normal formation and maintenance of bones and teeth .

If Deficient—In children, rickets (stunted bone growth, bowed legs, malformed teeth, protruding abdomen); in adults, osteomalacia (softening of bones leading to shortening and fractures, muscle spasms and twitching—adult rickets)

If Overdosed—Calcium deposits in soft tissues and excessive calcium in blood; general weakness, weight loss, nausea, loss of appetite, diarrhea; kidney damage (stones); high blood pressure

Vitamin E (Soluble in Fat)

Primary Sources—Vegetable oils; margarine; wheat germ; whole-grain cereals; bread; liver; dried beans; green leafy vegetables; asparagus; vegetable shortening

Main Roles—Reduces oxidation of vitamin A, the carotenes, and polyunsaturated fatty acids; aids in formation of red blood cells, muscles, other tissues

If Deficient—Deficiency is rare and difficult to cause experimentally; perhaps anemia and destruction of red blood cells

If Overdosed—No conclusive evidence; possibly muscle damage and fatigue

Vitamin K (Soluble in Fat)

Primary Sources—Leafy green vegetables; cabbage; cauliflower; peas; potatoes; liver; cereals; egg yolk; synthesis by normal bacteria in the intestines, except in newborns

Main Roles—Blood clotting

If Deficient—Hemorrhaging in newborn children, prolonged blood clotting time

If Overdosed—Jaundice in newborn children; an excess in adults is not likely

These four fat-soluble vitamins are stored in the body, so toxicity can be built up.

Vitamin C—Ascorbic Acid (Water Soluble)

Primary Sources—Citrus fruits; tomatoes; cantaloupe and other melons; green peppers; potatoes; dark green vegetables; cauliflower

Main Roles—Aids in formation of collagen, the connective tissue of skin, tendons, and bone; aids formation of hemoglobin; helps protect other vitamins from oxidation; helps in the absorption and use of iron and possibly protein and carbohydrates; may block the formation of cancer-causing nitrosamines

If Deficient—Scurvy (bleeding gums, muscle degeneration, weakened cartilage and capillary walls, skin hemorrhages, anemia); early symptoms are appetite loss, irritability, weight loss

If Overdosed—May cause destruction of B_{12} in ingested food; kidney and bladder stones; diarrhea; urinary-tract irritation; can cause dependency, especially in infants if taken by mother during pregnancy

Vitamin B_1—Thiamine (Water Soluble)

Primary Sources—Whole-grain flours; cereals; wheat germ; seeds such as sunflower and sesame; peanuts and pine nuts; legumes such as soybeans; organ meats; oysters; pasta; bread; peas; lima beans; might be in intestinal microbes

Main Roles—Necessary for carbohydrate metabolism

If Deficient—Beriberi (muscular weakness, swelling of the heart, leg cramps, constipation); need increases if caloric intake increases

If Overdosed—No known effect

Vitamin B_2—Riboflavin (Water Soluble)

Primary Sources—Liver; milk; kidney; cheese; eggs; leafy vegetables; enriched bread; lean meat; beans and peas; mushrooms

Main Roles—Helps release energy from carbohydrates, proteins, fats; aids maintenance of mucous membranes

If Deficient—Cracks at corners of mouth; scaly skin around nose and ears; sore tongue and mouth; itching and burning eyes; sensitivity to light

If Overdosed—No known effect

Vitamin B_3—Niacin (Water Soluble)

Primary Sources—Liver; poultry; fish; wheat germ; whole-grain flours and cereals; nuts; seeds; rice; peas

Main Roles—Along with thiamin and riboflavin facilitates energy production in cells; part of coenzymes necessary for hydrogen transportation and for health of all cells

If Deficient—Pellagra (skin rashes, especially on parts exposed to sun); diarrhea; sore mouth and tongue; depression and mental disorientation

If Overdosed—Flushing of skin; sometimes jaundice; duodenal ulcer; abnormal liver function; elevated blood sugar; possible gout

Vitamin B_6 (Water Soluble)

Primary Sources—Whole-grain cereals and breads; liver; meats; fish; poultry; potatoes; beans; brown rice; avocados; spinach; bananas

Main Roles—Especially involved in metabolism of protein; essential for conversion of tryptophan to niacin; helps body use fats

If Deficient—Skin disorders around eyes, mouth; sore mouth and smooth red tongue; weight loss; dizziness; nausea; anemia; kidney stones; nervous disturbances and convulsions

If Overdosed—Might lead to dependency

Vitamin B_{12} (Water Soluble)

Primary Sources—Only in animal foods: liver, meats, poultry, fish and shellfish; eggs; milk and milk products

Main Roles—Aids in formation of red blood cells; assists in building genetic materials; helps functioning of nervous system

If Deficient—Pernicious anemia (anemia, pale skin, new blood cells do not develop normally, and there is a deterioration of the spinal cord that can become irreversible); numbness and tingling in fingers and toes that could lead to loss of balance and weakness/pain in arms and legs. *Strict vegetarians at risk.*

If Overdosed—No known effects

Folacin (Folic Acid) (Water Soluble)

Primary Sources—Liver; leafy vegetables; wheat germ; dried beans and peas; asparagus; broccoli; nuts; fresh oranges; whole-wheat breads, cereals

Main Roles—Synthesis of nucleic acids vital to all cells; aids in formation of hemoglobin in red blood cells

If Deficient—Macrocytic anemia (red blood cells larger and fewer than normal); young blood cells do not mature; diarrhea

If Overdosed—No known effect

Pantothenic Acid (Water Soluble)

Primary Sources—Liver; eggs; wheat germ and bran; rice germ; peanuts; peas; widely distributed in most foods; also made by intestinal bacteria

Main Roles—Aids chemical reactions in body, particularly metabolism and release of energy from fat, protein, carbohydrates

If Deficient—Deficiency unlikely unless diet consists of highly processed foods and as part of deficiency of all B vitamins. Then symptoms include headache and fatigue; insomnia; abdominal stress; numb, tingling hands and feet; muscle cramps; loss of coordination and personality changes

If overdosed—No known effects

Biotin (Water Soluble)

Primary Sources—Egg yolk; liver; kidneys; dark green vegetables; green beans; widely distibuted in foods generally

Main Roles—Release of energy of carbohydrates; aids in formation of fatty acids

If Deficient—Scaly skin; mild depression; extreme weariness; muscular pains; highly sensitive skin; anorexia and nausea

If Overdosed—No known effects

Minerals

Calcium

Primary Sources—Milk and milk products; sardines, canned salmon (with bones); dark green leafy vegetables

Main Roles—Builds and maintains bones and teeth; muscle contraction (especially normal heartbeat rhythm); transmission of nerve impulses; proper blood clotting; enzyme activator

If Deficient—In children, rickets (stunted growth, retarded bone mineralization, poor bones and teeth, skeletal malformation); in adults, osteoporosis (brittle, porous bones)

If Overdosed—High levels of calcium in blood and urine, and in soft tissues; extreme lethargy; possibly kidney stones

Phosphorous

Primary Sources—Organ meats; poultry; fish; eggs, dried beans and peas; milk and milk products

Main Roles—With calcium, forms and strengthens bones; release of energy from carbohydrates, protein, fats; forms genetic material, cell membranes, many enzymes

If Deficient—Seldom in humans eating normal diet; weakness; bone pain; loss of bone calcium; poor growth

If Overdosed—Distortion of calcium-to-phosphorous ratio

Magnesium

Primary Sources—Leafy green vegetables; nuts; soybeans; seeds; whole grains

Main Roles—Release of carbohydrate energy; helps regulate body temperature, nerve and muscle contractions; helps adjust to cold weather

If Deficient—Deficiency occurs in alcoholics, people who eat highly processed foods, people who have prolonged diarrhea, kidney disease, diabetes, people who take diuretics; symptoms include weakness, tremors, dizziness, spasms and convulsions, delirium and depression

If Overdosed—Disturbed nervous system

Electrolytes

Potassium

Primary Sources—Widely distributed in foods; especially in oranges; bananas; cantaloupe; tomatoes; dark green leafy vegetables; liver; meat; fish; poultry; milk; bran

Main Roles—Release of energy from carbohydrates, protein, fats; with sodium regulates water balance, nerve irritability, and muscle contractions, including heart rhythm

If Deficient—Rapid heartbeat, heart failure; muscle weakness; nausea; kidney and lung failure; possible deficiency occurrence when doing hard work in heat

If Overdosed—Muscular paralysis; abnormal heart rhythms

Chloride (Chlorine)

Primary Sources—Table salt

Main Roles—Regulates balance of body fluids, acids, and bases as part of the fluid outside the cells; takes part in formation of gastric juices, absorption of vitamin B_{12}; suppresses growth of microorganisms in foods

If Deficient—Vomiting, diarrhea

If Overdosed—Disturbed acid-base balance

Sodium

Primary Sources—Table salt; MSG; soy sauce; baking powder; most other foods

Main Roles—Regulates water balance, muscle contractions, nerve irritability

If Deficient—Very rare; nausea; diarrhea; abdominal/muscle cramps

If Overdosed—High blood pressure (hypertension)

Trace Elements

Iron

Primary Sources—Liver; kidneys; red meats; eggs; leafy green vegetables; dried fruits; dried beans and peas; potatoes; blackstrap molasses; enriched and whole-grain cereals; *not in dairy products*

Main Roles—Transports and transfers oxygen in blood and tissues; part of hemoglobin in blood, myoglobin in muscles, protoplasm of cells, cell nuclei, and many enzymes in tissues

If Deficient—Anemia (red cells smaller, level of hemoglobin in them lower); faulty digestion; fatigue; shortness of breath

If Overdosed—Skin pigmentation; lowered glucose tolerance; cirrhosis of the liver

Copper

Primary Sources—In most foods, but especially organ meats, shellfish, nuts, dried beans and peas, cocoa; *not in dairy products*

Main Roles—Formation of red blood cells; formation of nerve walls and connective tissue; necessary for glucose metabolism

If Deficient—In some infants fed cow's milk (not breast-fed) can cause anemia; adult deficiency is unknown

If Overdosed—In Wilson's disease, a rare metabolic defect, there is abnormal storage in liver and other tissues which can cause uremia, heart defects, hypertension, violent nausea and diarrhea, death if not treated. *Cooking acidic foods in unlined copper pots can lead to toxic accumulations.*

Zinc

Primary Sources—Lean meats; fish; poultry; liver; eggs, dried beans and peas; wheat germ and bran; whole grains; milk

Main Roles—Constituent of insulin and enzymes important to digestion, protein metabolism, and synthesis of nucleic acids

If Deficient—Retarded growth (possibly "dwarfism"); retarded sexual development in children; anemia; poor wound healing; in prenatal children, abnormal brain development

If Overdosed—Nausea, diarrhea; fever; anemia; premature birth and stillbirth; bleeding in stomach

Iodine

Primary Sources—Iodized table salt; seafood; sea salt; *vegetables grown near the sea—persons living far inland from sea should use iodized table salt*

Main Roles—Regulates the rate at which tissues breathe oxygen

If Deficient—Tissues use less oxygen, the body slows down, and eventually so do the mental processes. Lack of oxygen results in goiter (enlarged thyroid with low hormone production); if mother has severe deficiency in first three months of pregnancy or before conception, cretinism in infants (retarded growth, protruding abdomen, swollen features, thick lips, enlarged tongue)

If Overdosed—If over extended period, could depress thyroid activity, also causing goiter

Fluorine

Primary Sources—Fluoridated water, natural or artificial; fish; most animal foods; foods grown in fluoridated water

Main Roles—Prevents tooth decay; may also be necessary with calcium and vitamin D to maintain strong bones and prevent bones from becoming brittle and porous in later life (osteoporosis)

If Deficient—Tooth decay in children; possible osteoporosis in adults

If Overdosed—Mottling of teeth enamel; deformed teeth and bones; a fatal poison in large doses

Chromium

Primary Sources—Meats; whole grains; corn oil; dried beans; peanuts

Main Roles—Metabolism of glucose and protein; synthesis of fatty acids and cholesterol; metabolizes insulin

If Deficient—Poor use of glucose possibly resulting in chemical diabetes and adult-onset diabetes

If Overdosed—Not known

Selenium

Primary Sources—Seafood; whole grains; meat; egg yolk; chicken; milk; garlic

Main Roles—As antioxidant, prevents breakdown of fats and other body chemicals; interacts with vitamin E

If Deficient—Not known in humans; in animals, degeneration of pancreas

If Overdosed—Not known in humans; animals suffer stiffness, lameness, loss of hair, blindness, death

Manganese

Primary Sources—Abundant in most plant and animal foods; whole grains; nuts; tea; instant coffee; cocoa powder

Main Roles—Synthesizes complex carbohydrates, fat, and cholesterol; functioning of central nervous system; normal bone structure; development of pancreas

If Deficient—Not known in humans; in animals, sterility and abnormal fetuses, bone deformation, muscle deformities

If Overdosed—Blurred speech; involuntary laughing; spastic gait; hand tremors

Molybdenum

Primary Sources—Legumes; cereal grains; liver; kidney; some dark green vegetables

Main Roles—Part of the enzyme xanthine oxidase

If Deficient—Not known in humans; in animals, decreased weight gain, shortened life span

If Overdosed—Loss of copper; goutlike syndrome

National Board of YMCAs. *The Official YMCA Fitness Program*. New York: Rawson Associates, 1984. Reprinted with permission.

D: GUIDE TO FAT IN COMMON FOODS

Choose more often			Choose less often
Low in fat Less than 15% of calories come from fat	**Medium** in fat 15-30% of calories come from fat	**High** in fat 30-50% of calories come from fat	**Very high** in fat Over 50% of calories come from fat

Vegetables & fruits

Fruits **Plain vegetables** (no added salt or fat) **Pure juices** Pickles* Sauerkraut*		French fries Hash browns	Avocados Coconut Olives*

*Prepared, canned, or frozen vegetables may contain salt or fat.

Breads & cereals

Grains & flours Barley Rice Bulgur Rye Corn Wheat Most breads Most breakfast cereals** Corn tortillas Grits Matzoh Noodles & pasta Popcorn (air popped) Rye wafers	Corn bread Flour tortillas Oatmeal Soft rolls & buns Wheat germ Plain crackers	Biscuits & muffins Granola cereals Pancakes & waffles Popcorn (popped in oil) Taco shells Snack crackers	Snack chips

*Most prepared products contain some added sodium from salt, baking powder, and baking soda. Salted crackers and chips are especially high, as are pancake and muffin mixes.

Dairy products

Nonfat (skim) milk Nonfat dry milk Dry-curd cottage cheese (unsalted) Sherbet**	Buttermilk* Plain lowfat yogurt Ice milk** Lowfat cottage cheese*	Lowfat milk (2%) Whole milk Creamed cottage cheese*	Butter Cream & sour cream Half & half Ice cream** Nondairy creamer Nondairy whipped topping **Most cheeses** Brie Cream cheese Cheddar Monterey Jack Gruyere Mozzarella Ricotta Neufchatel Swiss

cont.

Dairy products cont.

Low in fat	Medium in fat	High in fat	Very high in fat
			High-sodium cheeses
			Blue* American*
			Feta* Parmesan*
			Romano*
			Processed cheese products*

Protein-rich foods[1]

Beans & nuts

Low in fat	Medium in fat	High in fat	Very high in fat
Dried beans & peas		Soybeans	Tofu
Chestnuts			Nuts & seeds
Water chestnuts			Peanuts & peanut butter

*Packaged nuts and seeds may contain added salt.

Seafood

Low in fat		Medium in fat		High in fat	Very high in fat	
Cod	Abalone	Bass	Clams	Albacore	Anchovies	Shad
Flounder	Crayfish	Catfish	Crab	Carp	Herring	Trout
Haddock	Octopus	Smelts	Lobster	Salmon	Mackerel	Eel
Halibut	Scallops	Sturgeon	Mussels***	Tuna, drained of oil*	Sardines	Tuna in oil*
Perch	Sole	Fresh tuna	Oysters			
Seabass	Squid					
Shrimp***	Turtle					
Tuna in water*						

*Canned, dried, or pickled fish often contain large amounts of added salt.

Poultry

Low in fat	Medium in fat	High in fat	Very high in fat
Egg whites	Light meat of chicken & turkey (without skin)	Light meat of chicken & turkey (with skin)	Dark meat of chicken & turkey (with skin)
		Dark meat of chicken & turkey (without skin)	Duck & goose (with skin)
		Duck & goose (without skin)	Egg yolks***
			Whole eggs***

Meats

Low in fat	Medium in fat	High in fat	Very high in fat
Meats	**Completely trimmed**	**Completely trimmed**	**Partially trimmed**
	Beef round	Beef or veal	Beef or veal
	Veal (loin, round, or shoulder)	Lamb	Lamb
	Dried chipped beef*	Fresh ham or picnic	Pork
	Liver***	Cured ham or picnic*	Cured pork*
	Tripe	Kidneys***	**Completely trimmed**
		Heart***	Fresh pork loin
			Boston butt
			Ground beef
			Spareribs
			Veal cutlet
			Bacon*
			Canadian bacon*
			Cold cuts*
			Corned beef*
			Hot dogs*
			Brains***
			Tongue***
			Pastrami*
			Pigs feet*
			Salami*
			Sausages*
			Salt pork*

[1]Values are for cooked foods, prepared without added fat or salt.

cont.

Beverages

Low in fat	**Medium** in fat	**High** in fat	**Very high** in fat
Water	Buttermilk*	Lowfat milk (2%)	
Juices		Whole milk	
Nonfat (skim) milk			
Coffee (black)			
Tea (plain)			
Soft drinks**			
Beer, liquor, wine			
(moderation advised)			

Prepared foods

Spaghetti with tomato sauce	Shakes**	Beans & franks	Chili con carne
		Beef stew	Fried chicken
		Burrito	Hot dogs
		Cheeseburger	Onion rings
		Egg rolls	Potato chips
		Fried pork rinds	Snack chips
		Fish sticks	
		Fish sandwich	
		French fries	
		Frozen dinners	
		Hamburger	
		Lasagna	
		Macaroni & cheese	
		Pizza	
		Pot pies	
		Spaghetti with meat	
		Taco	
		Tamales	
		Tostada	

*Many prepared foods contain large amounts of added salt. Includes fast foods and other commercially prepared foods.

Condiments

Spices			Mayonnaise
Horseradish			Salad dressings
Tabasco sauce			
Vinegar			
Salt*			
Seasoned salt*			
Salted spices*			
Monosodium glutamate (MSG)*			
Catsup*			
Chili sauce*			
Pickles & relish*			
Soy sauce*			

*Many prepared seasonings and sauces contain large amounts of added salt.

Soups

Bouillons	Most soups	Cream soups	Cheddar cheese soup
Broths		Bean soups	New England clam chowder
Consomme			

*Most prepared soups contain large amounts of added salt.

Sweets

Sugar**	Caramel**	Most:	Chocolate (all types)**
Syrup**	Fudge**	Cakes**	Ice cream**
Honey**	Ice milk**	Cookies**	
Jams**	Pudding**	Doughnuts**	

cont.

Sweets cont.

Low in fat	Medium in fat	High in fat	Very high in fat
Jellies**		Pastries**	
Molasses**		Pies**	
Angelfood cake**		Candy bars**	
Fig bars**		Custards**	
Raisin biscuit cookies**			
Most hard candy**			
Mints**			
Marshmallow**			
Gelatin desserts**			

Fats & oils (100% of calories come from fat)

Choose more often

Polyunsaturated liquid oils	Liquid oils
Corn	Olive
Safflower	Peanut
Soybean	Stick margarine
Sunflower	Shortening
Soft margarine	Fat in chicken, fish, most nuts

Choose less often

Saturated
Butter
Lard & manteca
Coconut oil
Palm oil
Fat in beef, lamb, pork
Fat in dairy products

* = high **sodium** content; ** = high **sugar** content; *** = high **cholesterol** content

Note. Published with permission from "Eating for a Healthy Heart," a publication of The American Heart Association, Alameda County Chapter, P.O. Box 5157, Oakland, CA 94605.

E: CALORIE GUIDES TO EATING OUT

To help with your weight management goals when eating out, consult these typical menus from the five most popular kinds of restaurants: Mexican, Chinese, fast-food, Italian, and family-style. Numbers in bold typeface after the food item indicate its calories.

Mexican

Calories are relatively low for Mexican entrees, considering many are made with tortillas (pancakes) or tacos (crisp tortillas). Mexican salad plates and chalupas are especially low. The calories add up, though, if you start the meal with dozens of corn chips and Mexican dips and then add side dishes, a rich dessert, and wine to your order.

Appetizers

Nachos (tortilla chips topped with cheese and chili peppers), 5, **135**
Tostaditas (tortilla pieces or corn chips), 13 chips, **140**
Chili con Queso (melted cheese and pepper dip), ¼ cup, **180**
Guacamole (mashed-avocado dip), ½ cup, **210**
Ceviche (raw pickled fish), 3 slices, **240**

Entrees

Chalupas (fried boat-shaped shell filled with beans, cheese, lettuce), **95**
Chorizo (Mexican sausage), ½ cup, cooked, **170**
Chili (beef and bean), **180**
Tostada (open-faced corn tortilla with varied toppings), bean, **240**
Tamales (moist corn tortillas, filled, cooked in corn husk), beef, 2, **250**
Tortilla Casserole (ground beef, chili peppers, tomato, onion, cheese, tortillas), **250**
Quesadilla (flour tortilla filled with cheese, fried), **260**
Taco, beef, **260**
Enchilada (filled tortilla topped with sauce), pork, **275**
Taco, pork, **275**
Carne Asada (marinated beef), **300**
Chili Rellenos (batter-fried stuffed chilies), **300**
Arroz con Pollo (chicken with rice), **305**
Burrito (filled flour tortilla), chicken, **315**; beef, **360**; pork and bean, **380**
Chicken with Mushrooms in Sour Cream, **380**
Chimichanga (fried burrito), beef, **385**
Enchilada (filled tortilla topped with sauce), cheese, **390**
Tostada (open-faced corn tortilla with varied toppings), bean and beef, **400**
Huevos Rancheros (2 fried eggs on tortilla topped with tomatoes, green chilies, sour cream, avocado), **570**

cont.

Mexican cont.

Accompaniments

Salsa, green (tablesauce), ¼ cup, **55**
Tortilla, flour, **80**; corn, **85**
Spanish Rice, ⅓ cup, **90**
Refried Beans, 1 cup, **120**

Desserts

Buñuelos (fried pastries), 2, **130**
Sopaipillas (pastry puffs), 2, **160**
Flan (caramel custard), **335**

Beverages

Sangria, **155**
Chocolate con Leche (hot chocolate), **255**

Italian

With some preplanning and careful menu selections, Italian restaurants can still be among your eating out choices. Here are a few suggestions.

- Italian salad with dressing on the side, minestrone soup, and a side order of pasta served as the main meal are an ideal way to manage calories.
- Stay away from fried foods, anything filled or topped with a lot of cheese (lasagna, manicotti). Veal Piccata or Veal Scallopini Marsala are lower calorie choices.
- Pasta portions are apt to be generous. Leave some on your plate or have it as a smaller side dish with just a sprinkle of cheese.
- If you're going to have wine, order a single glass instead of a bottle or carafe.
- If you order dessert, share it and halve the calories.

Appetizers

Prosciutto, **65**
Mortadella, **90**
Clams Casino, **155**
Caponata (eggplant salad), **180**
Fried Zucchini, **195**
Tortellini in Cream Sauce, **510**

Entrees

Pizza, 1 slice, cheese, **150**; anchovy, **160**; mushroom, **160**; sausage, **200**
Breaded Veal Cutlets, **315**
Veal Scallopini (with lemon and butter), **340**

cont.

Italian cont.

Veal Scallopini Marsala (wine sauce), **340**
Veal Piccata (lemon and wine sauce), **375**
Beef Bracciole (rolled beef in gravy), **380**
Chicken Breasts with Prosciutto and Cheese, **435**
Eggplant Parmigiana, **470**
Veal Parmigiana, **520**
Chicken Cacciatore (chicken with peppers, onion, tomato, and wine sauce), **545**
Steak Pizzaiola (steak with tomatoes and anchovies), **690**
Risotto con Salaciccia (rice with Italian sausage), **770**

Soups

Minestrone, **200**
Escarole and Rice, **230**
Mussel, **375**

Pasta

Macaroni-twists, flat, shells, noodles, 1 cup, **155**
Spaghetti, 1 cup, plain, **155**; butter, **255**; tomato sauce and cheese, **260**; meatballs and tomato sauce, **330**
Fettucini Alfredo (wide noodles in cream sauce), **375**
Spaghetti Carbonara (bacon), **445**
Linguine with White Clam Sauce, **500**
Ravioli, beef, **500**; cheese, **550**
Lasagna, **630**
Manicotti (filled with cheese), **800**

Accompaniments

Sauteed Escarole with Garlic, **120**
Risotto alla Milanese (rice with Parmesan cheese and saffron), **230**
Zucchini with garlic and tomato, **240**
White Beans with Tomato and Garlic, **245**

Bread

Breadstick, **30**
Italian bread, **85**
Garlic bread, **120**

Desserts

Zabaglione (custard made with Marsala), **100**
Spumoni, **150**
Tortoni, **150**
Cheesecake, **300**

Beverages

Table wine (Chablis, Burgundy, Rhine, Chianti, rosé), **90**
Aperitif and dessert wines, sherry, port, Amaretto, Frangelico, Marsala, Madeira, **140**

cont.

Chinese

Chinese cooking is comparatively low in calories. Look on the menu for choices that are steamed, stewed, poached, or boiled. Add stir-frying to the list if you know the chef goes easy on the oil. Spareribs, dumplings, and deep-fat-fried dishes (like egg rolls) are obviously high in calories. There are still plenty of items to choose from: chicken-and-nut dishes, ones made with seafood, or slivers of meat tossed with tender-crisp vegetables. Even lo-meins (noodles) are a possibility if you eat a little less than a complete serving.

Appetizers

Crabmeat with Cucumber Salad, **40**
Shrimp Toast, 1 slice, **210**
Pork Dumplings (3), **270**
Egg Roll, **295**

Soups

Mustard Green, **30**
Egg Drop, **60**
Subgum, **75**
Bean Curd, **85**
Hot and Sour, **150**
Won ton, **190**

Entrees

Stir-Fried Bean Curd with Vegetables, **160**
Stir-Fried Scallops, **170**
Chicken Subgum (chicken and vegetables), **250**
Roast Pork, **265**
Egg Foo Yong, **270**
Steamed Chicken with Sausage, **270**
Pork with Broccoli, **290**
Sweet and Sour Shrimp, **290**
Batter-Fried Shrimp (5 large), **300**
Spicy Pork with Bean Curd, **345**
Chicken with Snow Peas, **375**
Sweet and Sour Pork, **385**
Striped Bass with Pungent Sauce, **390**
Chicken with Peanuts (or cashew nuts), **435**
Stir-Fried Chicken, **490**
Chicken Chow Mein, **510**
Moo Goo Gai Pan (chicken with snow peas, mushrooms, bamboo shoots), **540**
Chicken with Chestnuts, **560**
Chop Suey (with beef and pork), **600**
Fried Green Beans with Pork, **610**
Fried Rice with Chicken, **650**
Spicy Beef, **665**

cont.

Chinese cont.

Pork Lo-Mein, **670**
Barbecued Spareribs, **760**
Lobster Cantonese (with pork), **1145**

Accompaniments

Bean-Sprout Salad, **40**
Steamed Eggplant, **50**
Chilled Bean Sprouts and Cucumbers, **100**
Stir-Fried Broccoli, **105**
Steamed Rice, ½ cup, **110**
Noodle Salad, **130**
Sweet and Pungent Vegetables, **130**
Szechwan-Style Eggplant (in hot bean sauce), **160**

Desserts

Fortune Cookie, **35**
Kumquats (5 fresh), **65**
Almond Cookie, **135**
Chocolate Ice Cream, ½ cup, **150**

Beverage

Chinese Tea, **2**

Family Style

Entrees tend to be a little lower in calories in these restaurants because recipes are made with less rich ingredients: fewer eggs, milk instead of cream, etc. Stay away from breaded, fried foods, anything with piecrust or dumplings, and cream sauces. Waiters are used to taking special orders. Ask for foods baked or broiled instead of sautéed or deep-fat fried. Ask for butter, gravy, and salad dressings to be served on the side.

Soups

Consomme, **25**
Beef-Vegetable, **165**
New England Clam Chowder, **185**
Cream of Tomato, **215**
Lentil, **275**
Frankfurter-Bean, **285**
Split Pea, **290**

cont.

Family style cont.

Entrees

Fried Chicken, drumstick, **95**
Baked Flounder, **150**
Fried Chicken, ½ breast, **150**
Roast Turkey, **175**
Liver and Onions, **215**
Moussaka, **230**
Beef Pot Roast, **245**
Roast Beef, **245**
Chili con Carne (with beans), **260**
Chicken-Macaroni Salad, **270**
Meat Loaf, **280**
Chipped Beef (with cream sauce and noodles), **285**
Beef Stroganoff, **310**
Beef Stew, **320**
Grilled Steak, **330**
Creamed Eggs on Toast, **345**
Lasagna, **430**
Macaroni and Cheese, **430**
Swiss Steak, **435**
Spaghetti with Meat Sauce, **450**
Barbecued Brisket of Beef, **470**
Chicken a la King, **470**
Shepherd's Pie, **495**
Beef Pot Pie, **545**
Fried Pork Chops (floured), **570**
Chicken and Dumplings, **720**

Sandwiches

Chicken Salad, **260**
Egg Salad, **270**
Ham, **270**
Tuna Salad, **280**
Ham and Cheese, **300**
Roast Beef, **300**
Swiss Cheese, **340**
Bacon, Lettuce, Tomato (with one tablespoon mayonnaise), **360**
Grilled Cheese, **440**
Reuben (corned beef, sauerkraut, Swiss cheese), **550**

Accompaniments

Dill Pickle, **10**
Beets, **25**
String Beans, **25**
Mixed Green Salad, **40**

cont.

Family style cont.

Mashed Potato, **70**
Peas, **70**
Potato Salad, **125**
Coleslaw, **140**
French Fries (10), **140**
Baked Potato, **145**
Kidney-Bean Salad, **220**
Onion Rings, **350**

Desserts

Gelatin, **80**
Brownie, 1¾" by 1¾" by ⅞", **100**
Sponge Cake, **130**
Vanilla Ice Cream, **140**
Pound Cake, **140**
Chocolate Ice Cream, **150**
Chocolate Pudding, ½ cup, **190**
Tapioca Cream Pudding, **220**
Eclair, **240**
Coconut Custard Pie, **270**
Lemon Meringue Pie, **270**
Blueberry Pie, **285**
Cream Puff with Custard Filling, **300**
Apple Pie, **300**
Baked Custard, **305**
Boston Cream Pie, **310**
Cherry Pie, **310**
Lemon Chiffon, **355**
Devil's Food Cake, with icing, **365**
Cheesecake, **380**
Rice Pudding, with raisins, **385**

Fast Foods

Stick to the smaller, plainer foods: a hamburger instead of a deluxe cheeseburger, or a cup of chili instead of a chili dog. Unless you have an extra 300 calories or so to spare, pass up the french fries, frothy shakes, and desserts. Plan ahead and select a restaurant with a salad bar. Remember fast food doesn't mean you have to eat it fast.

Entrees

Hot Dog with bun, **273**
Scrambled Eggs, **180**

cont.

Fast foods cont.

Sausage (Pork), **205**
Chili, **230**
Fried Chicken (dark meat), **305**
Chili Dog, bun, **330**
Fried Chicken (white meat), **330**
Roast-Beef Sandwich, **350**
Chili Dog, with cheese, bun, **380**
Fish Sandwich (fried fish, sauce, bun), **390**
Cheeseburger, **307**
Hamburger, ¼ lb, **425**
Roast-Beef Sandwich with cheese, **450**
Hamburger, ¼ lb with cheese, **525**
Hot Dog, deluxe with cheese, **595**
Fried Clams, **615**
Pancakes with butter and syrup, **625**
Hamburger, double, **670**
Double Hamburger with cheese, **800**
Hamburger, triple, **850**
Triple Hamburger with cheese, **1040**

Accompaniments

Dill Pickle, **10**
Hash-Brown Potaoes, **125**
Coleslaw, **140**
Corn on the Cob, **175**
French Fries, small order, **250**
Onion Rings, breaded and fried, **300**
French Fries, large order, **350**

Desserts

Apple Pie or turnover, **255**
Cherry Pie or turnover, **260**
Strawberry Sundae, **290**
Cookies, **310**
Hot Fudge Sundae, **310**

Beverages

Coffee, **2**
Diet Soda, **2**
Tea, **2**
Soda, **95**
Hot Chocolate, **200**
Chocolate Milk, **215**
Vanilla Shake, **350**
Strawberry Shake, **360**
Chocolate Shake, **380**

Note. From "Clip-and-Save Calorie Guide to Eating Out" by C. Babigian, March, 1982, *Good Housekeeping Magazine*, pp. 68-72. Reprinted by permission.

F: CALORIE CHART

Fruits	Amount	Calories	Carbohydrate	Fat	Protein
Apple	1	61	15	0.6	0.2
Applesauce					
unsweetened	½ C	50	13	0.25	0.25
sweetened	½ C	116	30	0.15	0.25
Apricot	3	55	14	0.2	1
Avocado	½	188	7	19	2
Banana	1 medium	101	26	0.2	1
Blackberries	1 C	84	19	1	2
Blueberries	1 C	90	22	1	1
Boysenberries	1 C	88	22	0.2	2
Cherries	10	47	12	0.2	1
Cranberries	1 C	44	10	1	0.4
Dates	5	110	29	0.2	1
Fig, whole	1	40	10	0.2	1
Fruit cocktail					
in water	½ C	46	12	0.1	0.5
in syrup	½ C	97	25	0.15	0.5
Grapefruit	1	80	21	0.2	1
Grapes	10	18	4	0.3	0.3
Lemon	1	26	14	0.4	2
Lime	1	19	6	0.1	0.5
Mango	1	152	39	1	2
Muskmelon					
cantaloupe	½	82	20	0.3	2
casaba	1-2" wedge	38	9	Trace	2
honeydew	1-2" wedge	49	12	0.4	1
Nectarine	1	88	24	—	1
Orange	1	64	16	0.3	1
navel	1	71	18	0.1	2
Valencia	1	62	15	0.4	1
Florida	1	71	18	0.3	1
Papaya	1	119	30	0.3	2
Peach	1	58	15	0.2	1
Pear	1	100	25	1	1
Pineapple	1 slice	44	12	0.2	0.3
Plum	1	7	2	—	—
Prune	1	21	6	0.1	0.2
Pumpkin	½ C	41	10	0.5	1.5
Raisins	¼ C	119	32	Trace	1

Fruits cont.	Amount	Calories	Carbohydrate	Fat	Protein
Raspberries					
black	1 C	98	21	2	2
red	1 C	70	17	1	2
Strawberries	1 C	55	13	1	1
Tangerine	1	39	10	0.2	1
Watermelon	1 piece	111	27	1	2

Fruit Juices	Amount	Calories	Carbohydrate	Fat	Protein
Apple	½ C	51	15	Trace	0.1
Apricot	½ C	72	18	0.15	0.4
Cranberry	½ C	82	21	0.15	0.15
Grapefruit	½ C	48	12	0.1	0.5
Grape	½ C	84	21	Trace	0.25
Orange	½ C	61	14	0.1	1
Pineapple	½ C	69	17	0.15	0.5
Prune	½ C	99	24	0.15	0.5
Tomato	½ C	23	5	0.1	1

Vegetables	Amount	Calories	Carbohydrate	Fat	Protein
Artichoke	1 bud	12-67	15	0.3	4.3
Asparagus	4 spears	12	2	0.1	1
Bamboo shoots	½ C	41	1	—	0.3
Beans					
kidney	1 C	218	40	1	14
lima	½ C	106	20	0.2	7
snap	½ C	16	3	0.15	1
yellow/wax	½ C	14	3	0.15	1
Beansprouts					
cooked	1 C	35	7	0.3	4
uncooked	1 C	37	7	0.2	4
Beets	2	32	7	0.1	1
Broccoli	1 stalk	47	8	0.5	6
Brussels sprouts	4	30	5	0.3	4
Cabbage					
raw	1 C	22	5	0.2	1
cooked	1 C	31	7	0.3	2
Carrots					
raw	1	30	7	0.1	1
cooked	½ C	24	6	0.15	0.5
Cauliflower					
raw	½ C	14	2.5	0.1	1.5
cooked	½ C	14	2.5	0.15	1.5
Celery					
raw	1 stalk	7	2	—	0.4
cooked	½ C	11	2.5	6	0.5
Chickpeas	½ C	360	61	5	21
Coleslaw w/mayonnaise	½ C	87	83	9	1

Vegetables cont.	Amount	Calories	Carbohydrate	Fat	Protein
Corn	1 ear	70	16	1	3
creamed	½ C	105	26	1	2.7
whole kernel	½ C	87	22	0.5	2.6
Corn fritter	1 fritter	132	14	8	3
Corn grits	½ C	63	14	2.1	1.5
Cow peas	½ C	95	18	0.5	7
Cucumber	1	45	10	0.3	3
Eggplant	1 C	38	8	0.4	2
Kale	1 C	43	7	1	5
Lentils	½ C	106	20	Trace	8
Lettuce	1-3 leaves	2	0.4	—	0.2
Mushrooms	1 C	20	3	0.2	2
Okra	10 pods	31	6	0.3	2
Olives, green	10	45	0.5	5	0.5
Onion	1 T	4	1	—	0.2
Parsley	10 sprigs	4	1	0.1	0.4
Parsnips	1	106	24	1	2
Peas					
young	½ C	57	10	0.5	4.5
mature	½ C	115	21	0.5	8
Sweet peppers					
green	1	13	3	0.1	1
red	1	23	5	0.2	1
Pickles, cucumber					
dill	1	7	1	0.1	0.5
sour	1	7	1	0.1	0.3
sweet	1	51	13	0.1	0.2
Potatoes					
baked	1 large	145	33	0.2	4
boiled	1 medium	104	23	0.1	3
french-fried	10	137	18	7	2
hashed	½ C	178	23	9	2.5
mashed	½ C	69	14	1.25	2.2
scalloped					
w/cheese	½ C	178	17	10	7
w/o cheese	½ C	128	18	5	4
Radishes	10	14	3	0.1	1
Rhubarb					
raw	½ C	10	2.5	Trace	0.5
cooked (w/sugar)	½ C	191	49	0.15	0.5
Sauerkraut	½ C	21	5	0.25	1
Soybeans, mature, cooked	½ C	117	10	5	10
Spinach	1 C	14	2.4	0.2	2
Squash					
summer	½ C	15	3	0.1	1
Zucchini	½ C	13	3	2.1	2
winter, baked	½ C	65	16	0.4	2
Sweet potato	1 large	161	37	1	2

Vegetables cont.	Amount	Calories	Carbohydrate	Fat	Protein
Tomato	1	27	6	0.2	1
cooked	½ C	26	5	0.25	1
Turnips, cooked	½ C	18	4	0.15	0.6
greens	½ C	15	3	0.15	2
Vegetables, mixed	½ C	58	12	0.25	3

Cereals and Breads	Amount	Calories	Carbohydrate	Fat	Protein
Biscuit	1	103	13	5	2
Bran cereal	1 C	144	45	2	8
Cracked wheat bread	1 slice	66	13	1	2
French bread	1 slice	102	19	1	3
Vienna bread	1 slice	73	14	1	2
Sub roll	1 (11½ inches)	392	75	4	12
Italian bread	1 slice	83	17	0.2	3
Raisin bread	1 slice	66	13	1	2
Rye bread	1 slice	61	13	0.3	2
Pumpernickel	1 slice	79	17	0.4	3
White bread, enriched	1 slice	76	14	1	2
Whole wheat bread	1 slice	61	12	1	3
Bread stuffing					
cubes	1 C	111	22	1	4
dry	1 C	501	50	31	9
Cornflakes					
flakes	1 C	97	21	0.1	2
puffs	1 C	114	27	0.1	1
Corn bread	1 piece	161	23	6	6
Farina	½ C	52	11	0.1	2
Macaroni	½ C	78	16	0.3	2
Muffins					
corn	1	126	19	4	3
blueberry	1	112	17	4	3
bran	1	104	17	4	3
plain	1	118	17	4	3
Noodles					
egg	½ C	100	19	1	3
chow mein	½ C	110	13	5	3
Oatmeal	½ C	66	12	1	2
Pancakes					
buckwheat	1	146	17	7	5
plain	1	164	24	5	5
Rice cereal, puffed	1 C	60	13	0.1	1
Rolls/buns					
hard	1	156	30	2	5
hot dog	1	119	21	2	3
plain	1	83	15	2	2
roll	1	119	20	3	3
Waffles	1 section	140	19	5	5

Cereals and Breads cont.	Amount	Calories	Carbohydrate	Fat	Protein
Wheat cereal					
flakes	1 C	106	24	0.5	3
germ	1 T	23	3	1	2
instant	1 C	196	39	1	7
puffed	1 C	54	12	0.2	2
shredded	1 biscuit	89	20	0.5	3
Rice					
brown	½ C	116	25	0.5	2.5
white	½ C	112	25	0.1	2

Meat, Fish, and Fowl	Amount	Calories	Carbohydrate	Fat	Protein
Bacon	2 slices	86	0.5	8	4
Beef					
flank	3 oz	167	0	6	26
ground	3 oz	235	0	17	20
rib	3 oz	374	0	34	17
round	3 oz	222	0	13	24
rump	3 oz	295	0	23	20
sirloin	3 oz	329	0	27	20
Bluefish, baked/broiled	3 oz	123	0	4	20
Caviar	1 T	54	1	3	6
Chicken					
breast-roasted	½ breast	193	0	8	29
drumstick-roasted	1 piece	112	0	6	14
wing-roasted	1 piece	99	0	7	9
Clams	5	56	4	1	8
Codfish, broiled	3 oz	144	0	5	24
Crab	1 C	195	1	4	36
Fishcakes, fried	1	103	6	5	9
Fishloaf	1 slice	186	11	6	21
Fishsticks	1	50	2	3	5
Flounder	3 oz	171	0	7	26
Goose	3 oz	198	0	8	29
Haddock	3 oz	141	5	5	17
Halibut	3 oz	144	0	6	21
Ham croquette	1	163	8	10	11
Herring					
w/tomato sauce	1 fillet	97	2	6	9
pickled	1 piece	33	0	2	3
smoked	1 fillet	84	0	5	9
Kidney	1 C	353	1	17	46
Lamb					
leg	3 oz	237	0	16	22
loin	3 oz	341	0	28	21
rib	3 oz	362	0	32	18
shoulder	3 oz	287	0	23	18

Meat, Fish, and Fowl cont.	Amount	Calories	Carbohydrate	Fat	Protein
Liver					
beef	1 slice	195	5	9	22
calf	1 slice	222	3	11	25
chicken	1 liver	41	1	1	7
Lobster	1 C	138	0.4	2	27
Mackerel	3 oz	201	0	14	19
salted	3 oz	258	0	21	16
Oysters, cooked	4	108	8	6	4
Pig's feet, pickled	2 oz	113	0	8	10
Pork					
ham	3 oz	318	0	26	20
loin	3 oz	308	0	24	21
shoulder	3 oz	300	0	24	19
spareribs	3 oz	386	0	35	17
Rabbit	3 oz	176	0	8	24
Salmon					
pink	3 oz	155	0	23	7
broiled/baked	3 oz	156	0	6	23
smoked	1 oz	50	0	3	6
Sardines	1 fish	24	—	1	3
Sausage, cold cuts					
bratworst	1 link	172	0.4	15	7
bologna	1 slice	40	0.1	4	2
deviled ham	1 T	46	0	4	2
hot dog	1	176	1	16	7
headcheese	1 slice	76	6	4	4
knockwurst	1 link	189	2	16	10
liverwurst	1 slice	66	0	5	5
mortadella	1 slice	79	0.2	6	5
polish sausage	1	690	3	59	36
pork sausage	1 link	62	—	6	2
salami	1 slice	88	0.4	7	5
scrapple	1 slice	54	4	3	2
vienna sausage	1	38	—	3	2
Scallops					
fried	1	19	1	1	2
whole	1	29	2	1	3
Shrimp	10	37	0.2	0.4	8
Swordfish	3 oz	138	0	5	22
Tongue					
beef	1 slice	49	0.1	3	4
calf	1 slice	32	0.2	1	5
Tuna	½ C	158	0	7	23
Turkey	3 oz	215	0	13	22
light	3 oz	150	0	3	28
dark	3 oz	173	0	7	26
Veal					
chuck	3 oz	200	0	11	24
loin	3 oz	199	0	11	22

Meat, Fish, and Fowl cont.	Amount	Calories	Carbohydrate	Fat	Protein
rib	3 oz	229	0	14	23
round	3 oz	184	0	9	23
Venison	3 oz	107	0	3	18

Eggs	Amount	Calories	Carbohydrate	Fat	Protein
Fried	1	99	0.1	8	6
Hard	1	82	0.5	6	7
Poached	1	82	0.5	6	7
Scrambled	1	111	2	8	7

Dairy Products	Amount	Calories	Carbohydrate	Fat	Protein
Butter	1 t	34	—	4	—
Buttermilk	1 C	88	13	0.2	9
Cheese, natural					
blue/roquefort	1 ounce	104	0.6	8.6	6.1
brick	1 ounce	105	0.5	8.6	6.3
camembert	1 ounce	85	0.5	7	5
cheddar	1 ounce	113	0.6	9.1	7.1
cottage cheese					
w/cream	½ C	130	3.5	5	16.5
w/o cream	½ C	86	2.5	0.5	17
cream cheese					
regular	1 T	52	0.3	5	1
whipped	1 T	37	0.2	4	1
limburger	1 ounce	98	0.6	8	6
parmesan	1 T	21	0.2	1	2
swiss	1 ounce	105	0.5	8	8
Margarine	1 t	34	—	4	—
Milk					
whole	1 C	150	11	8	8
skim	1 C	88	13	0.2	9
lowfat	1 C	145	15	5	10
Yogurt, plain					
lowfat	1 C	123	13	4	8
whole milk	1 C	152	12	8	7

Beverages	Amount	Calories	Carbohydrate	Fat	Protein
Club soda	12 oz	0	0	0	0
Perrier water	12 oz	0	0	0	0
Cola	12 oz	144	37	0	0
Cream soda	12 oz	160	41	0	0
Fruit-flavored soft drink	12 oz	171	45	0	0
Ginger ale	12 oz	113	29	0	0
Root beer	12 oz	152	39	0	0
Diet drinks	12 oz	0	—	0	0
Cocoa powder, no milk	4 t	98	25	1	1

Beverages cont.	Amount	Calories	Carbohydrate	Fat	Protein
Coconut milk	1 C	605	13	60	8
Coffee	6 oz	2	—	—	—
Lemon juice	1 T	4	1	—	0.1
Lemonade	6 oz	81	21	—	0.1
Lime juice	1 T	4	1	—	—
Chocolate drink					
skim milk	1 C	190	27	6	8
whole milk	1 C	213	28	9	9
Hot chocolate	1 C	238	26	13	8

Alcoholic Beverages	Amount	Calories
Beer	8 oz	100
Eggnog, holiday variety, made with whiskey and rum	½ C	225
Whiskey, gin, rum, vodka		
100 proof	1 jigger (1½ oz)	125
90 proof	1 jigger (1½ oz)	110
86 proof	1 jigger (1½ oz)	105
80 proof	1 jigger (1½ oz)	100
70 proof	1 jigger (1½ oz)	85
Wines		
table wines (Chablis, claret, Rhine, and sauterne)	3 oz	75
dessert wines (muscatel, port, sherry)	3 oz	125

Sauces and Relishes	Amount	Calories	Carbohydrate	Fat	Protein
Catsup	1 T	16	3.8	0.1	0.3
Chili sauce	1 T	16	3.7	—	0.4
Horseradish	1 T	6	1.4	—	0.2
Jelly	1 T	49	12.7	—	—
Jams/preserves	1 T	54	14	—	0.1
Maple syrup	1 T	50	12.8	—	—
Mustard	1 t	4	0.3	0.2	0.2
Relish	1 T	21	5.1	0.1	0.1
Soy sauce	1 T	12	1.7	0.2	1
Tartar sauce	1 T	74	0.6	8.1	0.2
Tomato paste	1 C	215	48.7	1	8.9

Snacks and Desserts	Amount	Calories	Carbohydrate	Fat	Protein
Almonds					
unprocessed	12	85	3	8	3
roasted in oil	12	98	3	9	3
Cake					
angel food	1 piece	161	36	0.1	4
boston cream pie	1 piece	311	51	10	5

Snacks and Desserts cont.	Amount	Calories	Carbohydrate	Fat	Protein
chocolate					
w/o icing	1 piece	322	46	15	4
cupcake	1	121	17	6	2
w/icing	1 piece	365	55	16	5
cupcake	1	162	25	7	2
fruitcake	1 slice	57	9	2	1
gingerbread					
plain	1 piece	371	61	13	4
w/icing	1 piece	453	73	17	5
pound cake	1 slice	142	14	9	2
sponge	1 piece	196	36	4	5
white cake, w/icing	1 piece	386	63	14	4
yellow cake, w/icing	1 piece	365	61	13	4
coffeecake	1 piece	232	38	7	5
cupcakes					
plain	1	116	18	4	2
w/icing	1	172	28	6	2
devil's food	1 piece	312	54	11	4
Candy					
butterscotch	1 oz	113	30	1	—
caramels	1 oz	113	22	3	1
chocolate					
dark	1 oz	150	16	10	1
milk	1 oz	147	16	9	2
chocolate-coated nuts	1 oz	161	11	12	4
chocolate fudge	1 oz	122	21	5	1
candy corn	1 C	728	180	4	0.2
mints	10 pieces	64	16	0.4	—
gum drops	1 oz	109	28	0.3	0
jelly beans	1 oz	104	26	0.1	—
marshmallow	1	23	6	—	0.1
peanut brittle	1 oz	119	23	3	2
Cashews, roasted	18	159	8	13	5
Candied cherries	10	119	30	0.1	0.2
Chestnuts	10	141	31	1	2
Chewing gum	1 piece	5	2	—	—
Cookies					
brownies	1	103	15	5	1
butter	10	229	36	9	3
chocolate chip	10	495	73	22	6
coconut bars	10	445	58	22	6
fig bars	4	200	42	3	2
gingersnaps	10	294	56	6	4
ladyfingers	4	158	28	3	3
macaroons	2	181	25	9	2
marshmallows	4	294	52	10	3
molasses	1	137	25	3	2
oatmeal, w/raisins	4	235	38	8	3

Snacks and Desserts cont.	Amount	Calories	Carbohydrate	Fat	Protein
peanut	4	232	33	9	5
sugar wafers	10	170	26	7	2
peanut wafers	10	331	47	13	7
raisin	4	269	57	4	3
shortbread	10	374	49	17	5
sugar	10	355	54	13	5
vanilla wafers	10	185	30	6	2
Corn pudding	1 C	255	32	12	10
Crackers					
animal	10	112	21	2	2
butter	10	174	26	7	3
cheese	10	150	19	7	4
graham	1 cracker	55	10	1	1
sugar graham	1 cracker	58	11	2	1
saltines	10	123	20	3	3
soda	10	125	20	4	3
soup	10	33	5	1	1
Cream puff	1	303	27	18	9
Custard	1 C	305	29	15	14
Doughnuts, plain	1	164	22	8	2
Eclairs	1	239	23	14	6
Filberts	10	87	2	9	2
Fudge					
chocolate	1 oz	113	21	4	1
w/nuts	1 oz	121	20	5	1
vanilla	1 oz	113	21	3	1
w/nuts	1 oz	120	20	5	1
Gelatin					
plain	1 C	142	34	0	4
w/fruit	1 C	161	39	0.2	3
Grapefruit, candied	1 oz	90	23	0.1	0.1
Honey	1 T	64	17	0	0.1
Ice cream					
hard	1 C	257	28	14	6
soft	1 C	334	36	18	8
Ice milk					
hard	1 C	199	29	7	6
soft	1 C	266	39	9	8
Ices	1 C	247	63	—	1
Orange peel, candied	1 oz	90	23	0.1	0.1
Peanuts, roasted	10	105	4	9	5
Pecans	10	96	2	10	1
Pies					
apple	1 piece	302	45	13	3
banana	1 piece	252	35	11	5
blackberry	1 piece	287	41	13	3
blueberry	1 piece	286	41	13	3
butterscotch	1 piece	304	44	13	5

Snacks and Desserts cont.	Amount	Calories	Carbohydrate	Fat	Protein
cherry	1 piece	308	45	13	3
chocolate chiffon	1 piece	266	35	12	6
chocolate meringue	1 piece	287	38	14	6
coconut	1 piece	268	28	14	7
custard	1 piece	249	27	13	7
lemon chiffon	1 piece	254	36	10	6
lemon meringue	1 piece	268	40	11	4
mince	1 piece	320	49	14	3
peach	1 piece	301	45	13	3
pecan	1 piece	431	53	24	5
pineapple	1 piece	299	45	13	3
pumpkin	1 piece	241	28	13	5
raisin	1 piece	319	51	13	3
rhubarb	1 piece	299	45	13	3
strawberry	1 piece	184	29	7	2
sweet potato	1 piece	243	27	13	5
Rye wafers	10	224	50	1	9
Sesame seeds	1 T	47	1	4	2
Sherbert	1 C	259	59	2	2
Sunflower seeds	½ C	406	15	35	18
Tapioca pudding	1 C	221	28	8	8
Walnuts	10	322	8	32	7

Spreads and Salad Dressings	Amount	Calories	Carbohydrate	Fat	Protein
Blue/roquefort	1 T	76	1	8	1
low-calorie (5 cal/t)	1 T	12	1	1	0.5
French	1 T	66	3	6	0.1
low-calorie (5 cal/t)	1 T	15	2.5	1	0.1
Italian	1 T	83	1	9	—
low-calorie (2 cal/t)	1 T	8	0.4	0.7	—
Mayonnaise	1 T	101	0.3	11	0.2
Peanut butter (meat group alternative)	1 T	94	3	8	4
Russian	1 T	74	1.6	7.6	0.2
Thousand Island	1 T	80	2.5	8	0.1
low-calorie (10 cal/t)	1 T	27	2	2	0.1

Fast Foods[1]	Amount	Calories	Carbohydrate	Fat	Protein
Beverages					
Coco-Cola®	8 oz	96	24	0	0
Fanta Ginger Ale®	8 oz	84	21	0	0
Fanta grape®	8 oz	114	29	0	0
Fanta orange®	8 oz	117	30	0	0
Fanta root beer®	8 oz	103	27	0	0
Fresca®	8 oz	2	0	0	0
Mr. Pibb®	8 oz	95	25	0	0
w/o sugar	8 oz	1	Trace	0	0

Fast Foods cont.	Amount	Calories	Carbohydrate	Fat	Protein
Sprite®	8 oz	95	24	0	0
w/o sugar	8 oz	3	0	0	0
Tab®	8 oz	Trace	Trace	0	0
Hamburgers					
Burger Chef®					
Big Chef®	1	569	38	36	23
Hamburger	1	244	29	9	11
Super Chef®	1	563	44	30	29
Jack in the Box®					
Hamburger	1	263	29	11	13
Jumbo Jack®	1	551	45	29	28
Wendy's®					
Single	1	470	34	26	26
Double	1	670	34	40	44
Triple	1	850	33	51	65
McDonald's®					
Big Mac®	1	563	41	33	26
Hamburger	1	255	30	10	12
Quarter-Pounder®	1	424	33	22	24
Taco Bell® Bellbeefer®	1	221	23	7	15
Cheeseburgers					
Burger Chef®					
Cheeseburger	1	290	29	13	14
Double cheese	1	420	30	22	24
Jack in the Box® Cheeseburger	1	310	28	16	15
Jumbo Jack® w/cheese	1	628	45	32	35
McDonald's®					
Cheeseburger	1	307	30	14	15
Quarter-Pounder® w/cheese	1	524	32	31	30
Taco Bell Bellbeefer® w/cheese	1	278	23	12	19
Wendy's®					
Single w/cheese	1	580	34	33	34
Double w/cheese	1	800	41	50	48
Triple w/cheese	1	1040	35	72	68
Chicken					
Kentucky Fried Chicken®					
Original Recipe® dinner (drum and thigh)	1	643	46	35	35
Extra Crispy® dinner (drum and thigh)	1	765	55	44	38
Long John Silver's® chicken planks	4 pieces	457	35	23	27
Church's Fried Chicken®					
White chicken portion	1	327	10	21	23
Dark chicken portion	1	305	7	22	21

Fast Foods cont.	Amount	Calories	Carbohydrate	Fat	Protein
French fries					
French fries, average serving	1 pkg	220	26	12	3
Hot dogs					
Dairy Queen®					
Brazier® cheese dog	1	330	24	19	15
Brazier® chili dog	1	330	25	20	13
Brazier® dog	1	273	23	15	11
Super Brazier® dog	1	518	41	30	20
w/cheese	1	593	43	36	26
Super Brazier® chili dog	1	555	42	33	23
Ice cream, dessert					
Dairy Queen®					
Banana split	1	540	91	15	10
Chocolate-dipped cone					
small	1	150	20	7	3
regular	1	300	40	13	7
large	1	450	58	20	10
Chocolate malt					
small	1	340	51	11	10
regular	1	600	89	20	15
large	1	840	125	28	22
Chocolate sundae					
small	1	170	30	4	4
regular	1	290	51	7	6
large	1	400	71	9	9
Cone					
small	1	110	18	3	3
regular	1	230	35	7	6
large	1	340	52	10	10
DQ Parfait®	1	460	81	11	10
Dilly Bar®	1	240	22	15	4
DQ Sandwich®	1	140	24	4	3
Mr. Misty Float®	1	440	85	8	6
Mr. Misty Freeze®	1	500	87	12	10
Mexican food					
Taco Bell®					
Bean burrito	1	343	48	12	11
Beef burrito	1	466	37	21	30
Beefy tostada	1	291	21	15	19
Burrito Supreme	1	457	43	22	21
Combination burrito	1	404	43	16	21
Enchirito®	1	454	42	21	25
Pinto's N Cheese	1	168	21	5	11

Fast Foods cont.	Amount	Calories	Carbohydrate	Fat	Protein
Taco	1	186	14	8	15
Tostada	1	179	25	6	9
Jack in the Box®					
Regular taco	1	189	15	11	8
Super taco	1	285	20	17	12

Seafood

Burger Chef®					
Mariner Platter®	1 plate	734	78	34	29
Fish fillet	1	547	46	31	21
Dairy Queen®					
Fish sandwich	1	400	41	17	20
Fish sandwich w/cheese	1	440	39	21	24
Long John Silver's®					
Breaded oysters	6 pieces	441	53	19	13
Breaded clams	1 serving	617	61	34	18
Fish w/batter	2 pieces	366	21	22	22
Fish w/batter	3 pieces	549	32	32	32
Ocean scallops	6 pieces	283	30	13	11
Shrimp w/batter	6 pieces	268	30	13	8
McDonald's Filet O Fish®	1	432	37	25	14

Miscellaneous

McDonald's®					
Egg McMuffin	1	327	31	15	19
Buttered English muffin	1	186	30	5	5
Hot cakes, w/butter and syrup	1 serving	500	94	10	8
Sausage	1 serving	206	—	19	9
Scrambled eggs	1 serving	180	3	13	13
Apple pie	1	260	32	14	2
McDonaldland® cookies	1 pkg	308	49	11	4
Shake					
chocolate	1	383	66	9	10
strawberry	1	362	62	9	9
vanilla	1	352	60	8	9
Sundae					
hot fudge	1	310	46	11	7
caramel	1	328	53	10	7
strawberry	1	289	46	9	7
Burger Chef®					
Shake					
vanilla	1	380	60	10	13
chocolate	1	403	72	9	10

Note. Chart compiled from Adams, C. (1975). *Nutritive Value of American Foods, in Common Units* (Agriculture Handbook No. 456, USDA, Superintendent of Documents). Washington, DC: U.S. Government Printing Office.

[1]Reprinted with permission of Ross Laboratories, Columbus, OH 43216, from "Update: Nutritional Analysis of Fast Foods," *Public Health Currents* Vol. **21**, No. 3, 1981 Ross Laboratories.

G: REFERENCE SHELF

Checking It Out

Nutrition information comes from all sources these days—some reliable, others not. Because of the hundreds of new books and articles appearing each year on the topic of weight loss, it's especially important to be a nutrition-savvy consumer. To help judge the reliability of books and articles in newspapers and magazines, use this checklist.[1]

- What are the author's credentials?

  Is the author a registered dietitian or trained by a recognized university or college in an area relevant to nutrition? Remember, anyone can call himself or herself a "nutritionist," so take a critical look at the person's qualifications and professional affiliations.

- What are the author's sources?

  Nutrition is still a growing science and does not have all of the answers. Reliable writers will document their statements with references to the scientific journals that published the original research, and they will also indicate any evidence of conflicting research and unanswered questions. This documentation is especially important if the author is a journalist rather than a trained nutrition professional.

- Why was it published?

  Is the author or company tryng to sell you something? Is the author piggybacking his or her fame as an actor or athlete to sell his or her book? Interest in nutrition sells. Vitamin companies cannot make unsubstantiated claims; however, they can promote their products in magazines where such claims are made in "nutrition" articles and, thereby, indirectly influence sales.

- How is this information reviewed by nutrition professionals?

  The American Dietetic Association and Society for Nutrition Education publish nutrition journals that carry reviews on current nutrition books. The judgment of the nutrition department at your local college, university, health department, cooperative extension office, or dairy council office can also be helpful.

References

Use the following list of reliable references and resources on nutrition, health, and weight management to help put sound nutrition into practice.

Basic Nutrition Information

General nutrition and health:

A Diet for Living, Mayer, J., 1976. From Pocket Books, 1230 Avenue of the Americas, New York, NY 10020.

Jane Brody's Nutrition Book, Brody, J., 1981. From W.W. Norton & Company, 500 Fifth Avenue, New York, NY 10110.

Nutrition: Concepts and Controversies, Hamilton, E.M., and Whitney, E.N., 1979. From West Publishing Company, Box 3526, St. Paul, MN 55165.

Nutrition Cultism: Facts and Fictions, Herbert, V., 1981. From George F. Stickley Company, 210 W. Washington Square, Philadelphia, PA 19106.

Realities of Nutrition, Deutsch, R., 1976. From Bull Publishing Company, P.O. Box 208, Palo Alto, CA 94302.

The New Nuts Among the Berries, Deutsch, R., 1977. From Bull Publishing Company, P.O. Box 208, Palo Alto, CA 94302.

Vitamins and "Health" Foods, The Great American Hustle, Herbert, V., and Barrett, S., 1981. From George F. Stickley Company, 210 W. Washington Square, Philadelphia, PA 19106.

Food shopping:

Consumer's Guide to Food Labels, Food and Drug Administration, 1982. From Consumer Information Center, P.O. Box 100, Pueblo, CO 81002.

Eater's Digest: The Consumer's Factbook of Food Additives, Jacobson, M.F., rev. 1976. From Anchor Books, Doubleday & Company, 501 Franklin Ave., Garden City, NY 11530.

It's All on the Label, Understanding Food, Additives, and Nutrition, Block, Z., 1981. From Little, Brown and Company, Customer Service, 200 West St., Waltham, MA 02154.

What About Nutrients in Fast Foods?, Food and Drug Administration, 1983. From Consumer Information Center, P.O. Box 100, Pueblo, CO 81002.

Eating for Health and Weight Management

Healthy eating:

Food (1): A Publication on Food and Nutrition, U.S. Department of Agriculture, 1979. From Superintendent of Documents, U.S. Government Printing Office, Washington, DC 20402. (Stock no. 001-000-03881-8. Home and Garden Bulletin no. 228.)

Food 2: and *Food 3*: (two publications) *A Publication on Food and Nutrition*, 1982. From The American Dietetic Association, 430 N. Michigan Ave., Chicago, IL 60611.

Ideas for Better Eating: Menus and Recipes to Make Use of the Dietary Guidelines, U.S. Department of Agriculture, 1981. From Superintendent of Documents, U.S. Government Printing Office, Washington, DC 20402.

Nutrition and Your Health: Dietary Guidelines for Americans, U.S. Department of Agriculture and U.S. Department of Health, Education, and Welfare, 1980. From Consumer Information Center, P.O. Box 100, Pueblo, CO 81003

The American Heart Association Cookbook, 3rd ed., 1979. From Ballantine Books, 201 E. 50th St., New York, NY.

The Family Health Cookbook, White, A., and the Society for Nutrition Education, 1980. From David McKay Company, Two Park Ave., New York, NY 10016.

Weight Management and Low Calorie Cooking:

Diet Books Sell Well But . . ., Food and Drug Administration, 1982. From Consumer Information Center, P.O. Box 100, Pueblo, CO 81002.

Diets '81: Rating the Diets, Berland, T., 1981. From Consumer Guide, 3841 W. Oakton St., Skokie, IL 60076.

The American Diabetes Association and The American Dietetic Association Family Cookbook, Volumes I and II, The American Diabetes Association and The American Dietetic Association, Volume I (1980) and Volume II (1984). From The American Dietetic Association, 430 N. Michigan Ave., Chicago, IL 60611.

Facts about Obesity, U.S. Department of Health, Education, and Welfare, 1979. From Publications, National Institute of Health, Bethesda, MD 20014.

Lean Cuisine, Gibbons, B., and Consumer Guide, 1979. From Harper and Row Publishers, 10 E. 53rd St., New York, NY 10022.

Betty Crocker's Low-Calorie Cookbook, 1973. From Golden Press, New York, NY.

Better Homes and Gardens recipe books are available from Meredith Corporation, Consumer Book Div., 1716 Locust, Des Moines, IA 50336.

- *Calorie Counter's Cookbook*, 1983.
- *Dieting for One*, 1984.
- *Eat and Stay Slim*, 1979.
- *Low-Calorie Desserts*, 1972.
- *Low-Calorie Microwave Cookbook*, 1984.

[1]Adapted from Society for Nutrition Education. (1979). *Nutrition Information Resources for the Whole Family*, Berkeley, CA: Society for Nutrition Education.

Notes

138

Notes

Notes

Notes

Weight Graph

Weigh yourself once a week at the same time and place. Place a dot at a point opposite the total pounds lost for each week. Draw a line connecting the dots to see your progress at a glance.

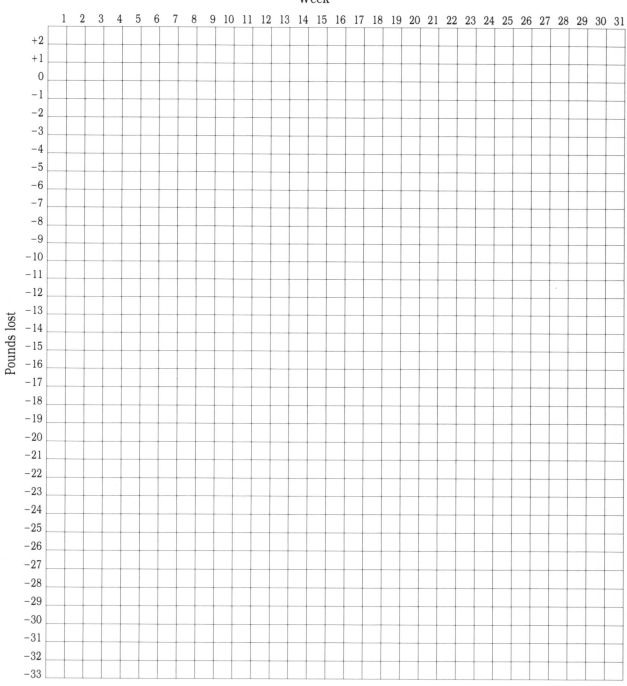

■ Y's Way to WEIGHT MANAGEMENT

Making a conscious commitment to managing your weight through diet and exercise is an important lifestyle decision. *Y's Way to Weight Management* teaches you the management skills and strategies necessary to achieve your diet and exercise goals. This personalized, action-oriented program gives you the current nutritional information you need to make intelligent daily food and exercise choices. Learning how to incorporate principles of weight management into your everyday routine will enable you to make a long-term commitment to a healthier, happier life.

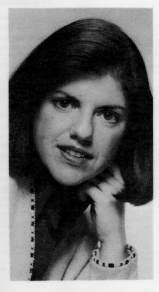

Registered dietitian and nutrition educator Sandra Konrad Cotterman heads the consulting firm Nutrition Communications® and is nationally recognized in the areas of program development and sports nutrition. Ms. Cotterman specialized in the area of weight management while on staff at Massachusetts General Hospital and has conducted hundreds of nutrition training programs for athletic, corporate, and consumer groups including the American Academy of Pediatrics, the American Dietetic Association, Junior Olympic Camps, the Boston Marathon, the U.S. Military Academy Army Athletic Program; and the U.S. Field Hockey Association.

Ms. Cotterman has been involved in developing national nutrition and fitness programs and recently served as project director for the Society for Nutrition Education's award-winning film on preschool nutrition. She received her B.S. in Dietetics and Home Economics Education from Purdue University, served a dietetic internship at Massachusetts General Hospital, and earned an M.S. in Nutrition and Communications from Boston University. She is a member of the American Dietetic Association, Society for Nutrition Education, and American College of Sports Medicine.

YMCA of the USA

ISBN 0-87322-032-3